# UNASHAMED

# Praise for *Unashamed*

'*Unashamed* is a pathbreaking psychological diagnosis of Indian society at a deep and fundamental level. It offers us ways and means to channelize our potential to be at harmony with ourselves and others in a constantly changing world. All of us, including our elders, need it as desperately as our youth to break free from the shackles of Colonial cultural mores. It's a guide to our true freedom.'

—**Aarti Tikoo Singh**, editor-in-chief, *The New Indian*

'Despite a dedicated effort over the last decade to produce much needed advancements in trauma and related issues, many individuals of our society are still uninformed or distressed. I applaud the author for writing *Unashamed*, a unique book that combines self-help and psychoeducation. It asks the reader a series of straightforward questions and challenges to help to reframe their views on relationships.'

—**Amitabh Bachchan**, actor

'I'm really looking forward to doing the work—it's about an aspect of my life that I definitely need help with and have constantly pushed away. Good luck to me! And you.'

—**Ira Khan**, CEO, Agastu Foundation

'We could all use a book like this. A step-by-step guide to recognizing shame and trauma in our bodies, and giving space for their expressions. The compelling questions and exercises at the end of each chapter are real, tangible tools in a journey to heal.'

—**Kalki Koechlin**, actress and writer

'*Unashamed* is sexual liberation, healing and cultural nuance, all in one.'

—**Leeza Mangaldas**, author of *The Sex Book: A Joyful Journey of Self Discovery*

'I enjoyed the book. This is a book that we all need to read to heal in today's time because trauma lives almost everywhere. I wish this book its best success.'

—**Nag Ashwin**, director and screenwriter

'If you are drawn to psychotherapy, you may find this book useful, as it addresses many sexualities in Indian contexts.'

—**Ruth Vanita**, author of *The Dharma of Justice in the Sanskrit Epics: Debates on Gender, Varna and Species*

# UNASHAMED

## Notes from the Diary of a Sex Therapist

## NEHA BHAT ATR-P

HARPER
NON-FICTION

First published in India by Harper Non-fiction 2024
An imprint of HarperCollins *Publishers*
4th Floor, Tower A, Building No. 10, DLF Cyber City,
DLF Phase II, Gurugram, Haryana – 122002
www.harpercollins.co.in

2 4 6 8 10 9 7 5 3 1

P-ISBN: 978-93-5699-628-1
E-ISBN: 978-93-5699-849-0

Typeset in 11.5/15.5 Adobe Garamond at
Manipal Technologies Limited, Manipal

Printed and bound at
Manipal Technologies Limited, Manipal

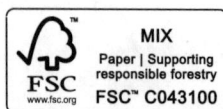

MIX
Paper | Supporting
responsible forestry
FSC
www.fsc.org
FSC™ C043100

This book is produced from independently certified FSC® paper to ensure
responsible forest management.

*To our inner guides,*
*whose voices we learn to repress*

The detailed references pertaining to this book are available on the HarperCollins *Publishers* India website. Scan this QR code to access the same.

# Contents

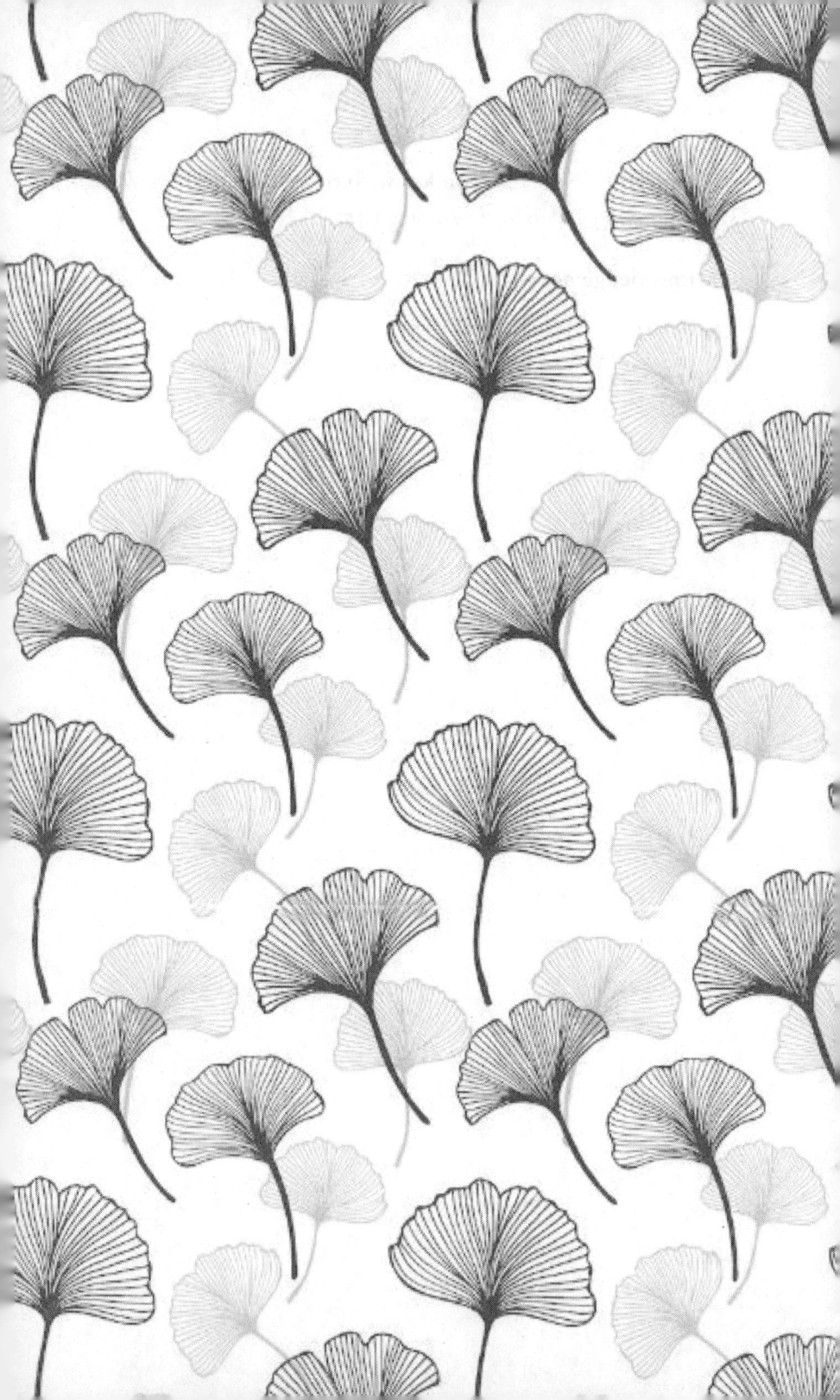

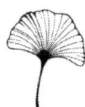

# PART 1

# Prepare

**_Why do we need to be unashamed?_**

_'Shame is the intensely painful feeling or experience
of believing we are flawed and therefore unworthy of
acceptance and belonging.'_

—_Dr Brené Brown, shame researcher and author of_
The Gifts of Imperfection: Let Go of Who You Think
You're Supposed to Be and Embrace
Who You Are _(2010)_

# Introduction

The rocks behind Bandstand in Bandra, Mumbai, hold a special place in my mind. As I write at my desk in my therapy office on a cloudy Wednesday afternoon, I'm reminded of the peculiar mix of sights and smells that dominates that unique place: dried papaya skin, sticky sweet sweat, salty air, fabric pressed against wet earth and slippery rock. In a morally-policed society like ours, where many of us are implicitly taught to live dual lives to avoid shame and judgement, these quiet rocks seem to offer honest solace for the city's lovers.

Passing by the sea, at first glance your eyes might perceive a blur of moving colour, intertwined body parts and shy laughter. You may naturally even want to turn away from the blur, sensing something intimate happening there. However, if you were to spend time by these rocks observing its many visitors at different hours of the day, you may hear the whispers of longing for unashamed intimacy.

You might find yourself surprised by the diversity of lovers in the mix here—from twenty-year-olds taking a break after college, watching music videos, sharing headphones and tiffin, to older couples nearing sixty stealing a quiet kiss, looking away if they happen to meet your eyes. The rocks serve as private spaces for the rest and play within a busy public maze. The privacy that this

3

space provides allows people from all sorts of backgrounds to have some respite from the challenges of our harsher Indian realities.

My name is Neha Bhat, and I'm a clinical sex-focused trauma therapist with trauma therapy training and practice, both, in India and the United States. I practice psychotherapy from a creative, art-based, multicultural lens. As a queer person, I care deeply about issues related to power, abuse and spirituality, in connection to collective health. I see value in simplifying complex, 'taboo' topics that can be hard to talk about, and in demonstrating how mental and sexual health are deeply connected—a bridge that has been waiting to be built for the Indian psyche.

My work has taken me to diverse places like urban and rural Karnataka, Maharashtra, Gujarat, Tamil Nadu, Kerala and New Delhi, as well as New York, Dubai, Paris, Amsterdam, Seoul and Chicago. During my fifteen years of practice, I have been humbled to witness the sexual–emotional realities faced by hundreds of people of Indian origin. In India, I have seen that the topic of sex and sexuality—from something as basic as the biological definition and what one's sexual and emotional needs are, to the more advanced inquiries of how to engage in a conscious manner and maintain joyful relationships over time—has been repressed or buried entirely. I identify this repression as a major cause of various forms of sexual trauma and mental dysfunction in our modern Indian psyche.

Living in a culture that hides key information about these topics causes layers of shame about what is supposed to be a natural part of human existence. Shame keeps people stuck in fear. And when people become fearful of their own biological needs, shame also causes us to look away from abuse and pain around those needs. Shame normalizes a culture of silence, secrecy and dysfunctional relationships. Healing gives people the power to change this.

A sex therapist's job is, essentially, to build alliances with people within their own realities. I play a dual role—of an observer and a teacher–advocate. The observer witnesses her client's challenges from a space of detachment, while the teacher–advocate invests energy in that person's difficulty to empower them to ease their own burden. Part of my life's work is to help people normalize their sexual and creative expression in relation to their personal power, to heal from sexual shame and expand their understanding of sexual trauma for a more joyful, balanced life. Therapy with a trained healing professional can help us heal from trauma and the trauma-based response, which is shame. Healing, as a process, gives us agency to then choose how we tackle our challenges.

During therapy sessions, there are two main types of questions I am asked by ordinary Indian people around the world. The first type tends to be about biology and body. These are topics which should have been taught at school: 'Is it okay for me to masturbate as a woman, man or trans-person?'(Yes, yes and yes!); 'Am I bad if I want to be touched by my wife in a way that feels good to me?' (Not at all, touch is a fundamental human need without which human beings cannot thrive); and so on. The second type of questions falls in the realm of emotional and relational health. These questions indicate how directionless we are about emotional maturity and wellness: 'Can I receive healing for the sexual abuse I went through as a child?' (Yes, and one must because the impact of childhood trauma often carries over into adulthood); 'Should I tell my husband about it?' (Yes please!); 'My partner won't talk to me for weeks after a fight—is this normal?' (No!); 'How can I ask my in-laws to give me more privacy at home?' (Let's help you develop better boundaries!); and other similar questions.

Normal, fundamental human needs have not only been made invisible but also been demonized by our complicated sociocultural history of colonial and religious trauma. A lack of social vocabulary around these topics in everyday life sees us struggle with questions and thoughts such as, 'How shall I tell my partner this?' or 'It's

so shameful to even want this or speak about this.' It is a major
factor that keeps shame—especially sexual shame—so alive in our
urban Indian lives and homes. We tend to believe in the myth that
marriage is a universal prescription—*shaadi ke baad khud pata
chal jayega* (you'll understand after you are married!). It should
automatically teach couples how to understand their own, their
partner's and their children's bodies, traumas, insecurities and
emotional needs. However, Indians are increasingly questioning this
script and wanting answers to their questions before any long-term
commitment.

As a diverse nation, India has unique realities not found anywhere
else in the world. Urban India is a melting pot of culture and religion,
and often two or three generations with different socio- political
values live together in joint families. In the overcrowded two-
bedroom apartments, sex and masturbation must be done silently
and without leaving a trace. In the middle of this intergenerational
conflict, we learn to have our emotional and sexual needs met while
causing minimal inconvenience to others. It is an unsaid expectation
in our country.

'Time will heal everything, just think positive for now' is a
common urban Indian adage especially heard at family gatherings
when the topic of someone's breakup, trauma or divorce comes up.
While time gives people the privilege of space to think, de-stress and
step away from the impact of one's pain, therapists all over the world
attest to the fact that time, by itself, cannot do anything. It has no
intrinsic healing power of its own. Healing from shame is a process,
a skill that has to be learnt—and that many Indians are hungry to
learn.

Through social media, more people are learning to name, frame
and speak to others about these very real human needs. Exploring
touch hunger, intergenerational conflict, urban isolation, porn

addiction and other less-discussed nuances of urban sexuality provides a lens for us urban Indians through which we can identify our own sexual histories of wounding and healing. Conversations (that urban millennial couples and families are having with each other) and podcasts, dating apps and TV shows targeted at these groups give us a glimpse of the giant waves of cultural change that are coming our way. As a society in flux, the changes will be seen even in the lesser-discussed areas of Indian life such as marital expectations, gender roles, mental health, emotional satisfaction, sexual desire and relational wellness.

While there is an information overload online, there aren't many practical, professional tools being offered to meet the intellectual, mental and emotional needs of the large number of urban Indians, who are trying to cope with these social changes in realistic ways. In this book, I've employed many case examples from my own therapy practice—of people's healing journeys from shame. The exercises after each chapter have been designed as self-help tools for sexual and mental wellness. I hope this book serves as a worthy companion as you choose to embark on this courageous path forward.

As India takes steps to improve facilities for its people, I sense that its social consciousness is ready to mature and evolve. The waves by Bandstand reminds me of the churning energy around me. This churn is how I make sense of our culture-in-transition presently. Unlearning generations of shame and shame-based trauma responses for a more liberated life is an act of courage. I believe it is time for us to invest in individual and collective trauma healing, because good health is a living, breathing possibility that each human being has a right to attain.

**Neha Bhat**
ABT, ATR-P
2024

# How to get the most of out of this book

Perhaps you're already in therapy and growing through it, or maybe you're someone who doesn't have the financial or social means to access therapeutic support. Perhaps you're sceptical and the social media buzzwords around trauma have piqued your curiosity. Or it could be that a recent relationship experience challenged your mental health and pushed you to read this book. Whatever your reasons are to be on this page, I applaud you for choosing to engage with this topic and wanting to learn about yourself.

This book has been designed as a therapeutic journey for understanding psychological complexities related to sexual shame in a step-by-step manner. It requires you to dig below the surface of narratives you might think of as 'obvious'. I've divided the book into four parts, each of which is focused on a separate step of a relational therapeutic journey. At the end of each chapter, I have provided a variety of exercises for practise from my professional therapy work.

It's important to remember that reading and writing about trauma isn't a replacement for trauma work with a trained mental health professional, who feels safe and consistent to you. No book can replace the presence of a human being. However, activities like creating art about our unspoken desires and longings, writing about our wounds to make them more cognizant, listening to music for relaxation, practising mindfulness for greater self-awareness, dancing, moving and telling our repressed stories in creative ways in trusted communities have immense therapeutic value. These activities can be called 'inner work tools'. I hope this book helps you create your own set of tools.

Any form of trauma work that includes deep reflection, exposing oneself to emotionally upsetting incidents, challenging ingrained patterns and invoking one's own creativity as a healing tool requires some basic sensitivity preparation first. You can, of course, choose to skip this part and dive right into the chapters, or you can read on to brace yourself a bit for this journey of inner work.

## Preparation Steps

### 1. Expect to 'sit with' your feelings for a long time

Throughout the experience of reading and processing the information and real-life narratives in this book, I urge you to 'sit with' the feelings that many uncomfortable, psychological and shock-inducing experiences, mirrored in this book, may bring up for you. Human beings are pain-avoidant creatures, and over time, we've developed many ways to avoid dealing with emotions that are difficult, complex and cause us physical or psychological discomfort. For example, imagine that you've just lost your pet to a car accident and are at a birthday dinner with your friend the next day. Your friend and you are talking about happy things like a comedy sketch or funny piece of gossip. As you eat your food, you suddenly start to remember your pet's warm touch. You feel your face getting warm and your chest starting to hurt. You cannot focus on what your friend is saying because your body hurts. When we feel the emotion of grief, it is a common experience to feel physical pain in the chest region, inability to speak and close to tears. Now, instead of taking a pause and accepting this feeling of incoming pain, you order a drink instead. Slowly, as the night progresses, one drink becomes two and two become four. Your body is now dealing with processing the drinks you've ingested to feel good. For now, you've successfully distracted yourself from feeling those painful sensations that the grief of death naturally brings up. You manage to have some fun that night, forget your pet's memory for a few hours and get a peaceful night's sleep. However, once you wake up the following morning, the chest pain has likely worsened and you feel like staying in bed and crying all morning.

When we avoid uncomfortable emotions, when we label them as 'negative' or view them as a punishment that we need to run away from, they tend to persist under the surface. Uncomfortable emotions act as a key to what may be unresolved and buried deep within us. The process of 'sitting with' feelings is about training our bodies to tolerate the short-term pain for a long-term gain. Learning how to handle the discomfort that complex feelings bring up, in the short-term, helps us let go of the emotion and resolve its overwhelming complexity in the long-term. Feelings become less burdensome when they are understood as a natural consequence of human life, are allowed to unfold at their own pace and are welcomed by our own selves, even in their messiness. This is what it means to practise 'sitting with' one's feelings.

While our feelings get lighter and simpler when they are welcomed and accepted, this should not to be mistaken for permission that all of our behaviours, too, need unconditional acceptance without accountability. Feelings and behaviours are different. For example, giving myself the permission to feel, accept and welcome my anger, my shame, my desire or my rage does not give me permission to act out these complex feelings on whoever is the easiest punching bag around me. I cannot physically or verbally harm someone and blame it on the side-effects of my inner work process. This would be a misunderstanding of inner work, while also being utterly irresponsible. Essentially, when we learn to practise riding the wave of our feelings of all types, we build pauses in our mind between the chain of action and reaction. These pauses give us the freedom to choose how we want to express the complicated and uncomfortable parts of us to those who care enough to listen.

Please remember that the process of 'sitting with' a feeling or a long set of feelings that are difficult and can initially feel very hard, even strangely counterintuitive, but this is exactly what creates deeper intimacy with ourselves. As you read on, you will find more tools for 'sitting with' your feelings in the following chapters.

## 2. Keep a small journal next to you

At the end of each chapter of this book, I've designed a few suggested exercises that can deepen your awareness. I invite you to keep a small journal with you as you read. A small, unused notebook in which you can write freely and move your hand across its pages should do perfectly well. See if you can maintain this journal throughout the completion of this book as you free-write your way through some of the chapters.

### 3. Learn to map what's happening in your body

Sometimes when we read something that connects to a very deep and likely tender part of our inner world, we can experience a variety of mixed sensations. On the one hand, it can feel liberating to finally find a word for that experience, but on the other hand, it can be an uncomfortable type of resonance. It can make you feel attacked, challenged, 'bad' or even slightly sad that you can now name that thing you do, or that feeling in your body you thought had passed. Shining a light on parts of our own sexuality that bring up physically complex feelings and that we might have had to stop paying attention to or have had to shut down is part of trauma work. If something feels too overwhelming to read, I suggest marking it down for another day and skipping ahead to a part that feels easier to digest. This is a non-linear process; there isn't one starting or finishing point, so start where your intuition takes you and find your own unique way of making this journey. Keep a glass of water close by as you take notes. Nourish your body if tears come out or you experience flashbacks or triggers.

### 4. Slow your reading pace consciously

In the age of social media, we're used to short, instant answers. Taking snippets of information from different sources. absorbing it all as one opinion and, then, regurgitating it on social media is one way to understand something. However, reading about something that has been demonized and hidden away inside us is, also, a powerful way to allow new thought patterns, new habits and new approaches to enter our system. As we do so, some resistance—or cognitive dissonance, which is something our minds do to protect us from information that challenges us to think differently—is expected and natural, because breaking one's inner conditioning is actually a complex matter of allowing our familiar inner stories and inner anchors to dissolve. So, don't feel daunted: please go as slowly as you need to. You might see yourself in some of these narratives—as some may strike very close to your own family patterns, sexual or romantic life—while you may find yourself utterly surprised by some others. All the case narratives are from real therapy experiences with my clients, reproduced with their consent. They are taken from clinical work, internships and community mental health therapy in different countries. Of course, personal details have been changed to retain anonymity.

## 5. *Share your reflections with a friend or a trusted person*

I suggest sharing parts of this book that feel relevant—a certain passage, a case example or, even, a psychotherapy term about sexuality that describes an experience you couldn't talk about before—with a trusted friend. You can then try to talk through what's being triggered in yourself. Talking through our lived experiences with people we trust is itself an anti-shame medicine. I want you to allow yourself the openness to *feel* through these words even as your mind exercises its rationality in understanding them. I also encourage you to discuss what you discover in this book through organizing a small meeting or a book discussion around it. Community can help us process the discomfort we might feel when we unearth taboos in a conscious, active, growth-oriented way. Undoing our individual and collective shame in groups of people we trust often helps us feel less alone and brings to light differences and nuances that help us steer away from being split into binary, rigid ways of seeing the world. It is exactly the type of shame-medicine that we Indians might benefit from more as we are part of a shapeshifting and complex society.

### 6. Set goals for your progress through this book

This book has been written with the intention of aiding you towards greater sexual and emotional maturity in this rapidly changing society, regardless of where you might be on your inner work journey. As you digest the chapters and work through the exercises, you might observe this book helping you in numerous ways. Here, I will help you name and map the starting point, since this is a challenging, shame-inducing and unfamiliar topic to deeply engage with.

### Goal 1

**Become emotionally more aware:** Building knowledge and awareness around our own behavioural patterns are parts of the first step towards this goal. How can you track your emotional awareness?

### Goal 2

**Experience deeper connection in your relationships:** Being trauma-informed may help you make sense of conflicting ideas, might teach you that two things can be true at once and we don't have to compete for there to be only one reality and only one form of truth. Trauma often teaches us about the hard realities of life, and coupling that with self-empowerment can bring you a sense of inner balance that helps when living in a paradoxical, complicated world filled with cultural and spiritual dissonance.

Being trauma-informed brings into our awareness where we may have not only experienced pain and hurt but also where we may have caused pain and hurt. We understand how the broken systems of our world actually maintain pain and hurt instead of trying to heal them. Mental health and sexual health are both important parts of our lives and deserve as much attention, if not more, as any other area of life healing.

Part of our traumatic, cultural conditioning as people healing from colonial trauma and other forms of oppression are toxic shame about sexuality, silence about sexual violence and unspoken intergenerational expectations about sexual desire. When we can bring awareness to the ways in which trauma kept the generations before us in silence, we can further understand our own shame—because shame is also a response to trauma in its own way.

### Goal 3

**Feel less alone in your life experiences:** With increasing urban development, many of us today have more physical resources than before. This could include things such as modern apartments, personal computers and fast internet. However, it is also true that more of us are feeling lonelier than ever. This is referred to as 'urban isolation'. I remember celebrating festivals in my childhood by gathering at the local park with our elderly neighbours. Today, the parks are scarce and playgrounds are often within gated communities. We, also, do not know too many of our neighbours.

As we expand towards becoming an economically stronger nation, our own city-based living realities have led to physical isolation, which has also seeped into the emotional realm. Urban isolation has caused more of us to view ourselves as solo sufferers of life's assaults. This is a sad myth that needs to be busted. We all seem to think we are especially unique and alone, when so many of our uncomfortable feelings and experiences are so culturally alike. Through the act of listening to the inner realities of others in Part 2 of this book, going deeper into your roots in Part 3 and then moving towards being shame-free in Part 4, you might feel relieved to learn that you're not alone.

## Goal 4

**Create your own inner work practices:** This book could also be used as an act of *self-permission*, allowing yourself the much-needed recourse to help alleviate shame, silence and self-judgement around sexual health that has been part of our Indian sexual conditioning. You can compile the tools you gain here with processes of soothing and support you might already know from other parts of your life. This innovation can then help solidify structures that work in favour of the unique circumstances of your life, helping you create your own trauma medicine, as explained in-depth in Chapter 10.

# A few trauma therapy terms used in this book

*Trauma:* Simply put, trauma is a type of wounding that causes distress. In mental health, it is defined as an emotional, psychological, mental or sexual response to events that are deeply distressing or disturbing to a person's sense of well-being. Trauma can happen at an individual level (sexual assault, for example) and at a collective, ongoing, systemic level (such as racism, casteism, religion-based discrimination and hate, misogyny and ableism). While there are many more complex and varied academic as well as clinical definitions of trauma, in my practice, I gravitate most towards renowned physician, Dr Gabor Mate's view as stated in his book *The Myth of Normal,* 'Trauma is not only what happened to you but it is also what happened inside of you as a result of what happened to you'. He states that trauma, in reality, is not the external event of the sexual abuse, the war, the parental neglect or the abandonment an individual or collective may have experienced. Rather, it is the internal wound that one carries forward from that experience. From the perspective of the Indian context, I find that this definition helps validate the often invisibilized experiences of many Indians who have been culturally conditioned to believe that they are somehow 'wrong' to feel upset, distressed and, even, traumatized by their life experiences, unless those experiences weren't extremely severe by nature.

There are further classifications used to distinguish between different levels of traumatic experiences based on their severity and impact. These terms help differentiate between events that are overwhelmingly distressing and events that are distressing but may not have as profound and lasting effects on an individual's psychological well-being.

*Big T Trauma*: Examples of 'big T' trauma include experiencing or witnessing severe accidents, sexual assault, natural disasters, hate crimes, war or other situations that may have led to death.

*Small t Trauma*: Examples of 'small t' trauma include experiencing bullying, divorce, loss of a pet, academic stress and interpersonal conflicts that cause disruption to one's regular life.

It's important to note that there is no clear-cut distinction between 'big T' and 'small t' trauma. Human beings respond differently to the same event depending on their individual well-being, resilience strategies and the support systems they had access to immediately after the traumatic event occurred.

*Buried Memory*: A memory that is hidden or repressed in a person's subconscious mind, often due to traumatic experiences. These are thought to be memories that the individual's mind has blocked from conscious awareness to protect them from the emotional and mental pain associated with the trauma that caused them.

*Trauma response*: How an individual's body, mind and spirit react to a traumatic or distressing event. Trauma responses are often both physical and psychological. During a fight, if your partner unknowingly uses a word to describe your behaviour that your father—who was perhaps a bully—used to insult your mother with, you might find your heart rate accelerating, your palms sweating and your voice getting louder until you burst into uncontrollable tears (physical response) and feel like your partner hates you or thinks less of you (psychological response). Trauma responses are ways the body and mind copes with the overwhelming stress and emotions associated with traumatic experiences. A few common types of trauma responses are:

1. **Fight, Flight, Freeze, Fawn**: These are the four well-known physiological responses to danger or threat. The body activates its stress response system, and we may feel an urge to fight back (fight), flee the situation (flight), become immobilized (freeze) or just give in to the threat so that it ends (fawn). These are explored in further detail in Chapter 6.

2. **Hyperarousal:** Being extremely vigilant of threat even when the cause of threat is not there, such as being unable to sleep after a traumatic event of physical assault. It can include experiencing flashbacks, intrusive memories and nightmares of the perpetrator of the trauma even when one is in a safer environment and being unable to relax weeks, months or years after the events have occurred. Intrusive memories are essentially fragments of trauma that suddenly intrude into an individual's thoughts and feelings. For example, a person could be in the bathroom getting dressed for a happy occasion when her mind recollects a physical assault that happened two months ago and she finds herself triggered and emotionally distressed.

3. **Hypoarousal:** Becoming emotionally numb or overtly detached and disconnected from yourself, your loved ones or your sense of purpose. The body creates this trauma response to reduce the intensity of distressing emotions.

4. **Avoidance:** When we consciously or unconsciously avoid people, places, activities or situations that remind us of the traumatic event to reduce our distress. For example, if you experienced bullying or a hate crime in college, you may never revisit it like others do or see it as a place of happiness. Your body might also want to keep you away from the relationships and people from the time of those traumatic experiences.

5. **Dissociation**: Experiencing a disconnection between different aspects of consciousness, memory, identity or perception. For example, you think you've been sitting at your desk trying to study for the past hour while feeling 'spaced out', but when you look at the clock, it's been six hours and you can't remember what you studied. A more extreme form of this would be when we are unable to locate where we are, what time of day it might be or what day of the week it is.

*Trauma-informed:* This is a worldview, an approach or a lens through which to look at health and wellness that acknowledges the impact of individual and systemic trauma in people's lives. It holds the view that all human beings are impacted by trauma and therefore seeks to create an atmosphere of understanding, respect and empowerment. Many schools, colleges, hospitals and workplaces are adopting trauma-informed practices to create a more inclusive, less harm-causing environment for people. This book explores how couples, families and close relationships of all kinds can benefit from adapting a more trauma-informed, compassionate lens.

This book is an extension of the conversations already happening around us. It is an offering of perspective on the intersections of mental health, sexual health and transitioning Indian culture in a depth-focused way. In my view, a book such as this could have helped Indian readers looking for support and perspective, and not finding it within their friends and families, during the impact of neoliberal American globalization of the 1990s.

Writing this book has been a tender yet activating process for me. Having learnt to navigate the many aspects of my own queer sexuality within the Indian context, teaching myself the very therapeutic skills and techniques I share with you to find your own answers to some complex questions between culture and future and having witnessed in client after client, the resilience that flowers when one engages with inner work practices, I can safely say that the fruits of inner knowledge are worth the work one puts in. I hope you will find yourself mirrored in some of the reflections here and call into yourself the capacity to live a more heart-centered, unashamed and creative existence.

Let's dive right in.

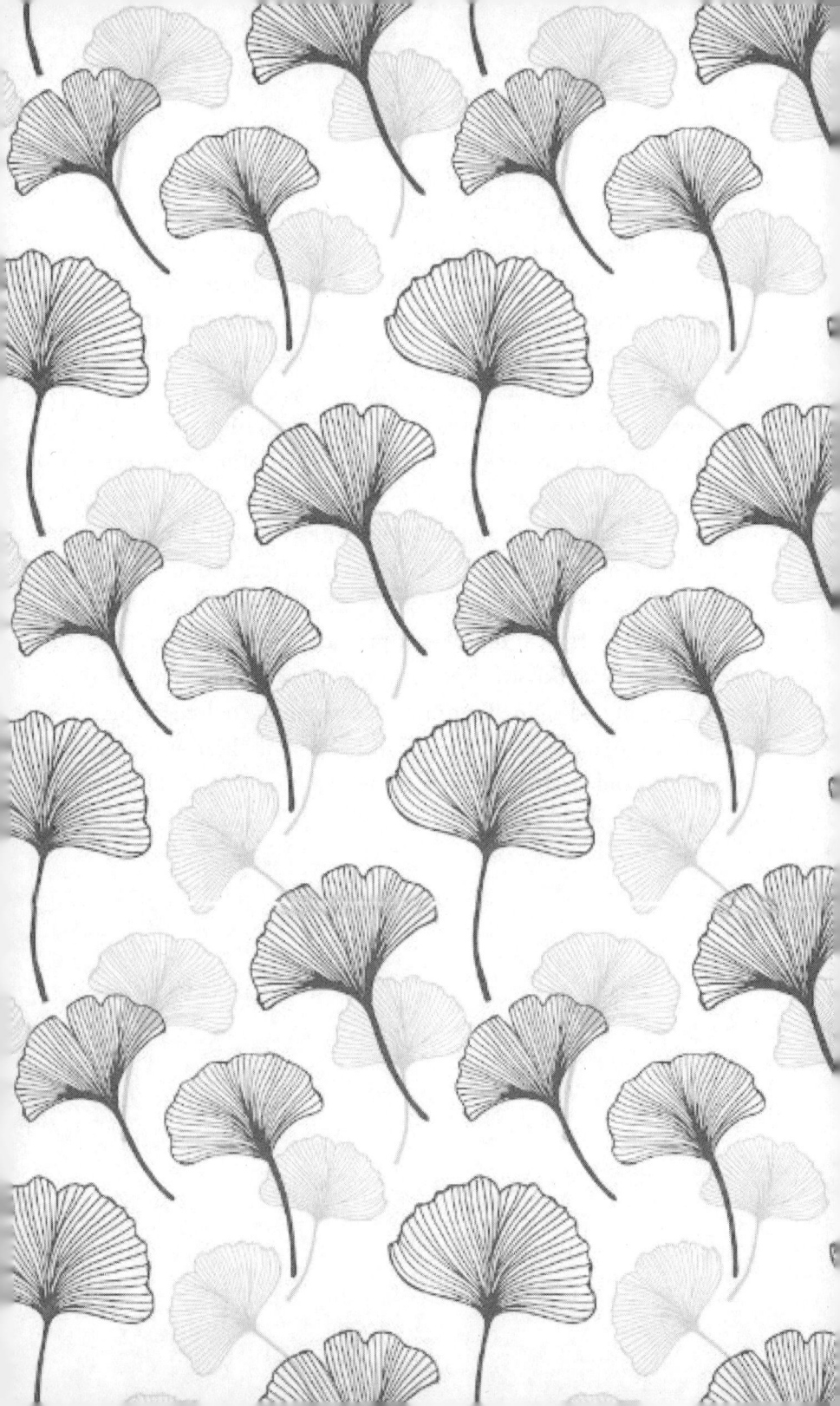

# PART 2

# Listen

## What's our shame trying to say?

*'Just as in family therapy, the first stages of a client's growth happen when denial and minimization are reduced, when persons can go more deeply into the layers of defense that cover their interior feelings. When congregations peel off the outer cloak of everything being "just fine" and look at the wounds they carry, it will be painful.'*

—Karen A. McClintock, *trauma-informed psychologist*

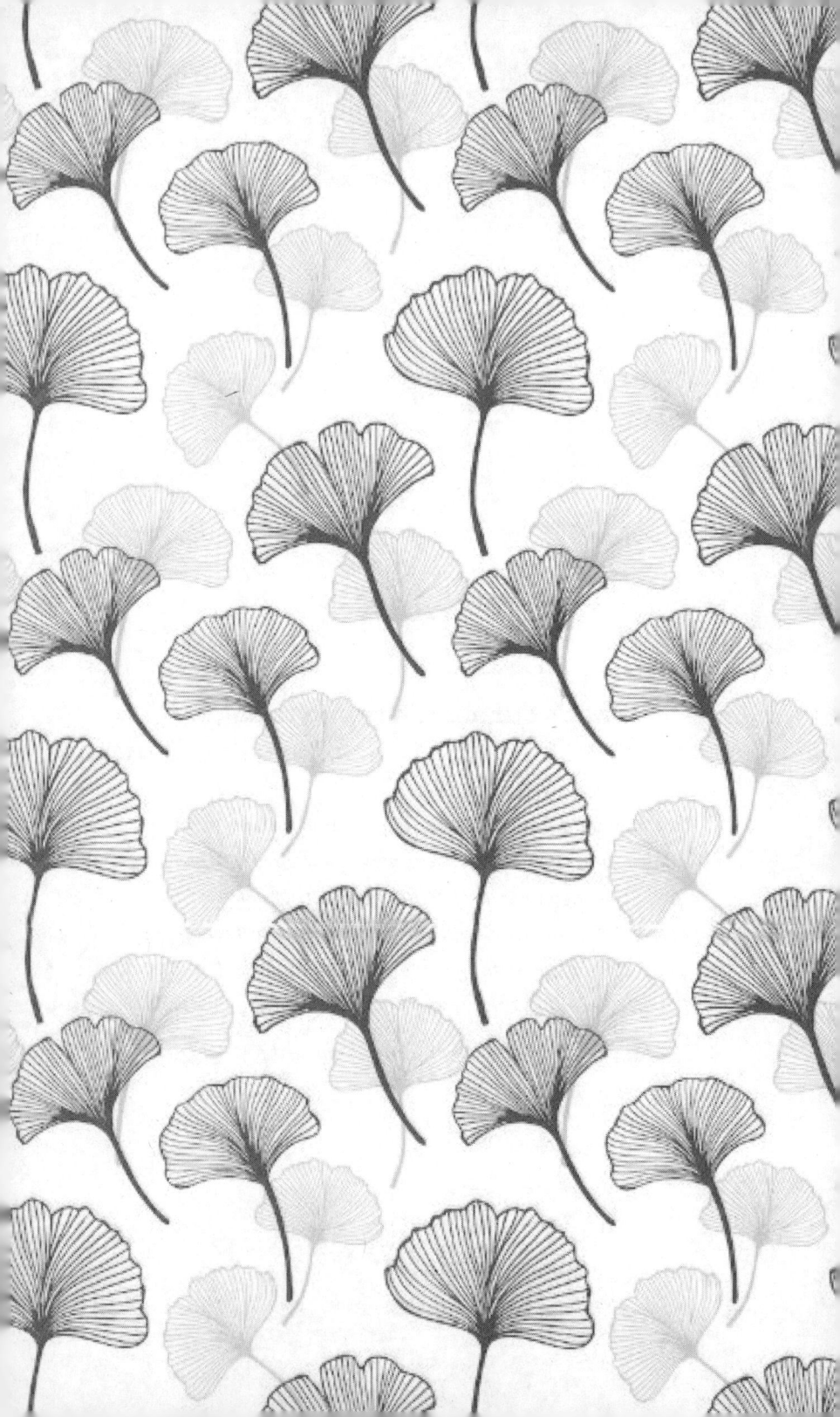

# CHAPTER 1

# 'Why do I feel shame in my body, even when I long deeply for sexual touch?'

## *On desire and shame*

Kusha came into my therapy office on a blistering Sunday afternoon with what felt to me like a large metaphorical 'suitcase of repressed sexual shame'. The sun's heat seemed to match the fiery rage with which she entered our therapeutic alliance that day. 'Ever since I started masturbating at fourteen—and I know I started later than most girls—a deep, intense feeling arises in my body as soon as I start feeling good,' she told me. 'When I try to describe it to you, it feels like a sad feeling—but I think it is more intense. It feels like it is trying to hide somewhere, because it doesn't like itself and doesn't want to be seen. When I orgasm, I feel this sad feeling more. It seems as if this feeling has a life of its own and its life is not in my control. When I listen to my friends discuss their sex lives, I feel a sort of burning rage inside me. I know I can have that type of carefree happiness too—I want it badly—but it doesn't happen. I don't understand why I can't get this sadness to stop. I want to feel good touching my body, Neha, but I can't—I don't.'

When she spoke, Kusha would say she was sad, but as I listened to her narrate her experiences, in my body, I started to sense a quiet anger coming from her. In each session, as I allowed my own body to sit with these somatic senses (feelings my body was taking on from her, as we say in somatic work), I would gently bring these feelings to her attention by asking, 'Do you notice that there's some anger here, present in the room right now, Kusha?' I would bring attention to her clenched jaw as she would sob or her tight fists squeezing her handkerchief and ask, 'What would it feel like if we gave it some attention?' I remember the visceral feelings in my body each time she would leave my office after therapy. I would want to go for a walk or a run, to release the energy I'd taken on from her.

Four sessions in, and as she got more comfortable in our alliance, Kusha revealed that she was angry with everyone in her life for being better than she was. She had always been judged as 'too intense', 'too talkative' and 'too loud'. At thirty, she was witty, fiery and blunt with her words, and exhibited a passionate desire to understand herself better. To this day, Kusha has been one of my only patients who was ready to unpack her 'suitcase of rage' without me even asking her to open it.

Kusha could be described as a woman with a lot of energy who had been asked to quieten down over the years by all those who loved and cared for her. The solitary walks I would take after our sessions would bring my attention to how much Kusha carried around in her own body, how much feeling had been repressed and how much of her anger she had learnt to mask as sadness. It would feel as if her nervous system had been carrying buckets of extra energy for years—an excess she did not know how to spend.

'I remember the advice I received about sex, sexuality, consent and boundaries as a child,' she said. 'If you like him, say "no". Let him work a little harder to get to you.' She was told that at thirteen by her mother. Kusha said that her parents were open-minded and had brought her up 'with as much freedom as an average Indian parent would give a son'. They valued education above getting married and having children and so she was permitted to read, write and think about what she liked, unlike a lot of families in her neighbourhood.

'What do you mean by "permitted to", Kusha?' I asked. At first, Kusha seemed frustrated at my explorations of her history. She insisted that her 'childhood was actually fairly comfortable and ideal' and it was just that her 'body, for some strange reason, was broken', because of which she could not experience physical pleasure without feeling intense shame. Was there a hormonal problem, she asked, or perhaps a sex toy I could recommend so that she could move on from all this and finally feel good?

'Kusha, I am so sorry,' I said, gently, one session after she circled back to these questions. 'I'm sorry you haven't been feeling in control of your own body, desire and experience. It must be so frustrating to hold that present truth, to accept it and to stay with it. I wish issues around our sexualities could be solved by simply inserting a sex toy and ending all our frustrations with ourselves, but it just isn't how our complex systems work. Despite what the sex-positive advertising sirens tell us, a simple toy does not help us understand the roots of our shame. We are a mix of so many internal truths and external lies, there is much to uncover. Help me help you go deeper, would you? What's beneath this feeling for you—this pain of not being in control of your physical experience?'

Sometimes, hearing me say this or a version of it, Kusha would become physically very still, trying to sit with what her therapist was asking of her. Something about these words and the tone I used would melt her heart. On other days, her anger with herself—and then with me, for not prescribing the perfect sex toy—would act as a block for her to see anything else for some time. She would fixate on what a broken person she was, and how everyone else was much better off than she could ever be. Her shame spirals were stubborn patterns that would take over and make her loud and angry at my words.

However, being the well-read, articulate person Kusha was, her angry outbursts would soften after a few minutes and she would feel further ashamed about not knowing that her rage could overtake her, even in therapy. And so, she would close her heart back up and steer our conversations to other topics as a way to deflect from sitting with her intense feelings. She once said that virginity was a social construct, and I agreed. We talked about how our teachers at school had explained virginity as a hymen-based biological phenomenon, when in fact the hymen can break during cycling, yoga or any other form of exercise. Penetration, or putting something inside you, cannot and absolutely does not define your worth.

I proceeded slowly. Session by session, Kusha unpacked compartment after compartment of her 'rage suitcase', finding new boxes to open each time. Once, as we were exploring the cultural shame of being told she was ugly by her school friends because she was not light-skinned, she suddenly came upon a deeply repressed memory. This changed the trajectory of therapy for Kusha. 'Neha … I remember someone watching me change my clothes. I … can almost see him in my mind right now,' stuttered Kusha. 'How old are you in this memory, can you tell?' I asked. 'I think I'm a child … about seven …'

In this memory, Kusha was seven years old. Her parents had taught her to always be aware of her surroundings while she was changing her clothes, to ensure that the curtains of her room were drawn and her privacy protected. One afternoon, as she was changing out of her school uniform, listening to the radio and getting ready for skating class, she thought she saw an older man's face peeping inside her bedroom through her window. As she focused her gaze on the window, she made eye contact with him. With her naked seven-year-old body trembling in utter fright, Kusha screamed loudly, making her mother rush to her bedroom. Kusha said she could not remember what happened after that.

Kusha and I both experienced this moment as profoundly moving in the therapeutic process. I could tell something of immense importance had been uncovered because Kusha was uncharacteristically quiet. Her hands were shaking, her breath short and shoulders tense and scrunched up. Working through this traumatic experience was going to cause pain because after being pushed underneath the surface, it had now seen the light of day—but in the presence of a trusted person.

I could also tell that words weren't going to be enough since that traumatic moment was still present in Kusha's adult body. 'Would you like to let your hands speak, Kusha?' I asked. She quickly agreed. I guided Kusha to allow her memory to take the form of a free drawing on paper, as she entered a *hypoaroused freeze response* (more on this later) from having chanced upon this buried memory (see page 19) in therapy. It was from this point on that we began to experience a radical shift.

Depictions of healing on television generally cut to a sense of relief and a 'healed' feeling when TV characters experience shapeshifting moments like this with their TV therapists. This is not how healing works in reality. For some time after this point, Kusha started experiencing rawer feelings of shame, anger, pain and grief. As she allowed those hidden parts of her to see daylight again, she started learning how to let her body create more space inside to contain them. Her gaze had become cold towards those hidden parts, and she had to teach herself to be warm and tender towards them.

As it so happens in therapy, when we give access to one buried, unseen need of ours through gentle, warm self-acceptance of that need, a lot of interconnected needs and feelings receive permission then to take solid form. It's like feelings speak to each other like children and wait for turns to be shown attention by a secure adult. From being forgotten and intangible, they start to become tangible and grow. Often, because we have had no connection to these old, hidden parts of us, our own bodies can feel overwhelmed by the growth and intensity of our new experiences and feelings, until we teach ourselves patiently to accept its new growth. This is what inner work practice is all about.

Kusha slowly started to make the connections between the assaultive, penetrating impact of the man's gaze on an unsuspecting child's naked body and her body's deep need to protect itself with layers of masks—which is what shame is. Shame is a protective mechanism, a mask. Her body had been trying to protect her all along!

'So, Neha, you're telling me that this intense feeling of shame I experience when I masturbate is connected to this experience? Isn't that just crazy? I thought time eventually heals everything,' Kusha said. And in the next moment, she closed her eyes and wept for the rest of that session.

Over time, Kusha internalized the truth behind what she learnt about her own shame. She had discovered for herself through allowing her body to experience those complex old feelings and not being afraid of them that she had actually been deeply impacted by that older man's perverted gaze. At the time, she was a child, who is not yet supposed to be in control of their physical experience. Like all children, she was in an innocent body feeling safe in the confines of her own home, and a strange adult had broken this feeling of safety and shocked her child self. Her body was naturally going to feel afraid.

Seven-year-old Kusha had felt so terrified when she found a stranger watching her undress that her body had produced a scream of terror at that moment. This scream met two purposes if we analyse it deeply: one, it notified her parents that she was in danger and needed help. Kusha had essentially been assaulted without being touched in an incident that had breached the safety of her own bedroom. And two, we could consider that the scream also created a signal for Kusha's own body that she was experiencing something intense—something that made this child feel helpless, something that her body could not control.

'What happens when you can't control something?' I asked Kusha. 'Think of a teacher who can't control her class, or a boss who can't get their employee to do their job.'

'You fire the employee, or you yell at your students to listen to you,' replied Kusha.

'Precisely.'

When the body has no way to control an experience and that experience creates a huge shock—such as sexual trauma—the body tries to shut that experience down so that it can stay safe and be 'in control' again. 'Could it be, Kusha, that your shame is actually your body's way of protecting you from something you didn't have the ability to process, remember or understand?' I asked. 'Could it be that that feeling of sexual shame you experience is a residue of the body's very old, unprocessed fear of losing control?'

Shame can be seen as a form of fear (see page 34). It took Kusha some gentle sitting with her pain to really see the protective function of the very feeling she hated in herself. She learnt to undo keeping her feelings and needs small, buried and repressed. Slowly, under her own healing gaze, she learnt to replace the memory of the assaultive gaze of her perpetrator.

Each time she felt shame as she experienced pleasure, she reminded herself that her body just needed reassurance from her to accept the good feelings of pleasure that she was receiving. She was an adult now. This gave her access to her own body, her own heart and her own inner GPS that she could learn to trust. She was in the driver's seat now. As an adult, she could redirect her shame with practise, guidance and self-compassion.

What she had gradually uncovered through therapy was that the very shame she hated when her body experienced pleasure was the same unconscious medicine her 'broken' body had produced to keep her safe from the memory of that horrible assault all those years ago. Unlike her perpetrator, who had tried to receive pleasure from the body of a child who could not consent to participating in a sexual relationship of any sort, she no longer needed to carry that fear of pleasure as her self-protection. Even though our wounds can feel like heavy burdens to carry, they often teach us about resilience and strength. Kusha slowly learnt to stop punishing herself for feeling good, and after her inner work process, she was able to embrace her shame while integrating it into her sexual health practices.

The nature of sexual violence is such that it is passed on from one person to the other through the dynamics of abuse. Many perpetrators of sexual violence have experienced sexual violence at some point in their lives, and sometimes survivors of sexual violence also perpetrate that same violence on others. Yet there are many, many individuals who experience severe trauma but who never go on to harm others.

The connections between abuse and pleasure and fear and shame are made early in life, somewhere between childhood and adolescence. The feelings of shame and anger—which naturally happen as a consequence of the abuse—can become mixed up with sexual feelings, leading to confusion in the person who experienced the abuse. This is what Kusha experienced and punished herself for. She assumed it was her body's fault when it absolutely was not.

Our feelings of inadequacy and helplessness can get buried deep within our sexual, emotional 'suitcases' and we can, like Kusha, often forget about them until we are confronted with an unrelated life circumstance with a 'familiar pull'. Then it's time to gently unpack them one by one with ample self-compassion and courage.

*'Her shame was a wound that would eat itself. Like lemon juice dripping on burnt skin, she would feel good punishing herself for what she thought was her "being bad".'*

Notes to myself in my art therapy journal, after one rainy afternoon session with Kusha.

## Chapter Takeaways

Sexual abuse is unfortunately common, and can have lifelong consequences. The painful feelings of shame and anger—which develop naturally as a consequence of being abused—can sometimes become mixed up with sexual feelings even after the trauma has ended, leading to debilitating confusion in the person who experienced the abuse. When we educate ourselves about the psychological, cultural and social realities of sexual trauma, instead of staying ashamed and silent about it, we can understand and organize the complexities living inside of ourselves better. This helps us enhance the quality of our individual and collective lives.

# Exercise 1: Reflect

*This reflection exercise is designed to help you assimilate the key points touched in this chapter. Once you finish reading the list of terms below, please fill in your answers below each question.*

**Trauma:** Some clinicians and researchers define trauma as a singular distressing event or a set of distressing events that causes shock to a person, place, animal or unit's sense of wellbeing. Others define trauma in a less specific and more encompassing way. They see trauma to be a response to events that cause extreme stress, sometimes on an ongoing basis.

**Traumatic:** something that causes deeply distressing trauma.

**Traumatization:** the act of inflicting trauma

**Shame:** the uncomfortable and painful sensation we feel when it seems we are consumed by judgement, either by others or by our own selves for doing something, saying something or being a certain way.

**Sexual shame:** the inherent feeling that one is 'wrong' or 'bad' for feelings, desires or actions related to sex and sexuality. Sexual shame is learnt, it is not in-born. Cultural messages, religious trauma, movies, negative judgements, bullying messages and poor awareness of fundamental human needs and realities can cause sexual shame. Sexual shame can be overcome and sexuality can be embraced and enjoyed with self-acceptance, validation, and appropriate sexual and mental health education.

## Reflection Questions:

1. What does the word 'trauma' mean to you in your own life?

.................................................................................................

.................................................................................................

.................................................................................................

.................................................................................................

.................................................................................................

.................................................................................................

.................................................................................................

.................................................................................................

.................................................................................................

.................................................................................................

.................................................................................................

.................................................................................................

.................................................................................................

2. What was the most surprising, intriguing or challenging part about this chapter for you? Why was it so?

.................................................................................................

.................................................................................................

.................................................................................................

..............................................................................................................

..............................................................................................................

..............................................................................................................

..............................................................................................................

..............................................................................................................

..............................................................................................................

..............................................................................................................

..............................................................................................................

..............................................................................................................

..............................................................................................................

..............................................................................................................

## Exercise 2: *Learn to 'sit with' your uncomfortable feelings*

After reading about Kusha's narrative in Chapter 1, you may feel unsettled, intrigued, triggered, charged, activated or simply interested in going further. These are all perfectly healthy, natural responses to ingesting information about a topic as evocative and all-pervading as sexual assault and its connection to sexual desire. It's important to remember that grounding yourself can help ease your feelings. Our reactions, however upsetting, can be beautiful reminders of our humanity. Learning to create awareness and space for our reactions within our own body is essential to tolerating our own distress.

Keep your writing material close to you as you immerse in this somatic reflection.

- Find a supportive place for your legs. It could be the ground, a bed or any hard surface. Make sure your lower body is supported.

- Close your eyes and place your hands on your belly.

- Breathe in as deeply as you can as you count upwards. On the count of seven, hold your breath for five counts and then breathe out as slowly as you can till the count of seven (this is belly breathing).

- Think of the words 'shame' and 'body'. Imagine them flashing in the centre of your mind's eye, taking shape, form, colour, maybe even a smell.

- What images, thoughts, feelings or sensations surface for you? In what ways does Kusha's narrative impact you? Stay with this question for as long as you can.

- When you notice your body getting tired of holding attention to this prompt, gently hold your pen and allow your hand holding the pen to freely move on the paper in front of you.

- Try to allow whatever is arising to flow, to be, without any self-judgment of what it may mean. It could be art, it could be music, it could be words that someone has said to you or something you believe about yourself—the form is irrelevant here.

- Stop when you feel done; please don't push yourself beyond your capacity.

- Spend five minutes in silence after.

Some people feel like crying when they practise 'sitting with' themselves. Others feel irritated, cranky, overwhelmed and restless. All these responses are okay. By practising grounding, you will learn how to be mindful when you are distracted by feelings that threaten to come out of hiding in a big way. The aim is to learn how to ride the waves of emotions, sensations, triggers and irritations as and when they come without getting drowned by them. This will feel hard when you start, especially because culturally we are conditioned to 'move on' from big feelings by our families and romantic relationships.

Other than going to an ashram or attending a religious ceremony, we may not know how to bring an inner stillness to our somatics in our everyday life. When you are habituated to not attending to your big feelings, you might become numb to them over the years. That stored trauma then releases itself in other, indirect ways that can hurt others and yourself. This is why people are surprised when they have huge emotional outbursts weeks, months or years after an incident and then they often do not know the source of their feelings.

When I feel really angry, for example, instead of intellectualizing how I should not get angry, or calling a friend to distract me from my anger, I take myself on a walk. I do this exercise of 'sitting with' myself for about five minutes and tell myself, 'Neha, you're going to feel this emotion intensely for the next half an hour.' In that period, I walk near my office or sit at the local park, allowing my nervous system to process what's coming up without shame or inner judgement. Nine times out of ten, after I complete this exercise I have trouble remembering why I was so angry when I started.

I like to remind myself that pain in this life is not avoidable, but the pain we create in trying to avoid pain is avoidable. If you're currently working with a therapist, it might be a great idea to take this material into personal therapy and see where this takes you in your own process of understanding yourself and your specific relationship to the world.

# Exercise 3: Build a relationship with yourself through writing

Your feelings and sensations are your body's voice and language— they are the only ways your body can speak to you. Every day, we navigate our complex world and its harsh systems using our body. In a way, our body is our own complex, intelligent GPS system – it shows us the way in silent ways. A lot of us also live in disconnection with the very bodies that house us, sometimes without even knowing that this might be the case.

One of the big ways shame hurts us is by making us think, 'When I feel bad, it means I am bad.' Shame is judgemental and has lofty expectations. Shame doesn't know how to distinguish between feeling, thought, action and behaviour; it mixes them all in one big sensation. When we aren't used to listening to our body's sensations, we also aren't used to understanding what it might be trying to tell us.

Writing is a process of making the intangible, tangible. By its very nature, the act of writing for oneself involves trying to listen to what one's inner voice wants to say. The process of freewriting can feel liberating. It can allow us to channel our sense of truth underneath all the confusing messages our bodies pick up from the world, show us patterns we weren't aware of and help us make sense of them in a concrete way.

Freewriting can uncover memories we didn't know we could access and can help us sort through complicated life situations by bringing up surprising insights. It can also give us an opportunity to be honest with ourselves and this can feel especially healing if we have trouble doing so. Freewriting is a portal towards authenticity because it can quickly help parse through the buildup of everyday muck that blocks our connection to that depth inside of us.

There is no one right method of freewriting. The process has freedom in its very name, so the point is to try and write as openly, as fearlessly, as unabashedly as possible, in the safety of your own gaze. Many schools of thought also call this 'stream of consciousness writing', signifying that the writer allows thoughts, emotions, feelings, hidden memories, flashbacks and names of people, places and events to freely flow like a river without a beginning or an end.

Let's begin. Please start with the same initial steps as described on page 37. Grounding ourselves is pivotal to any experiential exercise which has the potential to go deep.

- Find a supportive place for your legs. It could be the ground, a bed or any hard surface. Make sure your lower body is supported.
- Keep your journal close to you.
- You can choose to play music of your liking as you're getting comfortable.
- Keep your favourite writing tool close to you. I like fountain pens with blue ink as my brain associates them with clear feelings. You are free to choose a colour pencil, a sketch pen, a gel pen or a ballpoint pen—any writing tool that you find easy and comfortable to hold.
- Close your eyes and place your hands on your belly.
- Breathe in as deeply as you can as you count upwards. On the count of seven, hold your breath for five counts and then breathe out as slowly as you can till the count of seven.
- Slowly open your eyes, take your pen and with large, easy strokes, write whatever comes to your mind. It can be in any language and can be curse words or taboo words, insults or

compliments. Don't judge or think too much. Don't worry about grammar or punctuation. The sentences can stop erratically and start at a different point. Like art, paint with your pen freely. Don't read what you're writing just yet.

- Stop after about ten to fifteen minutes.
- Stretch your body and start again. I like to take my clients through this start and stop process a few times until they feel comfortable being 'in the zone' and not judging what they're doing.
- Once you decide to stop, put your pen down and gently massage your body where it's stiff after sitting for so long.
- Gently observe what you wrote in the last fifteen minutes.

Now, ask yourself the following questions:

1. Are there any patterns, repeated words, feelings, thoughts or emotions that I'm noticing in my freewriting pages today? If so, what were these?

.......................................................................................................................

.......................................................................................................................

.......................................................................................................................

.......................................................................................................................

.......................................................................................................................

.......................................................................................................................

.......................................................................................................................

.......................................................................................................................

........................................................................................................

........................................................................................................

2. Did I notice any parts of my body tense up when I was writing a particular sentence?

........................................................................................................

........................................................................................................

........................................................................................................

........................................................................................................

........................................................................................................

........................................................................................................

........................................................................................................

........................................................................................................

........................................................................................................

........................................................................................................

3. Were there parts of my body that felt relaxed when writing specific words or thoughts?

........................................................................................................

........................................................................................................

........................................................................................................

........................................................................................................

........................................................................................................

........................................................................................................

..................................................................................

..................................................................................

..................................................................................

..................................................................................

Spend five minutes writing these answers down, then write the date on the pages. Please remember to limit the time you spend doing this. If you want to free write for five minutes, stop at five and not thirty. People who are disconnected from their body's language tend at first to convert a physical experience into a solely mental one. This is counterproductive to learning to listen to the language of your body.

Now, please close the process for yourself. If you're intellectually driven, you might be tempted to analyse everything you've written and make sense of it. If you're more driven by feelings, you may not want to get into it. I would suggest letting freewriting be free. After you close the process for the day, restore your journal to its safe space where no one else can access it. When you return to it the next time, you might notice that you have new reflections or insights about what surfaced for you.

Many people who freewrite regularly make it a part of their morning ritual. This is when their subconscious is the most open to being in a relaxed flow state, just before the demands of the day. Kusha liked to freewrite at night before sleeping. It helped channel her rage at the flaws of the world that her body experienced so intensely and helped her sleep better as well.

# CHAPTER 2

# 'What's all this hullabaloo about therapy and isn't inner work just woo-woo?'

*On embracing inner work practices without shame*

'What really is therapy?' is a common question I get asked at Indian dinner parties when I answer the generic, 'So, what do you do?' and reveal that I'm a psychotherapist. While the word is popular in certain sections of urban Indian society, it is still very much a practice shrouded in mystery and vagueness within our mainstream. Therapy is a professional form of inner work. Let's first define the broad category of 'inner work' and 'inner work practices' and then proceed to understanding what therapy is.

Professional occupations such as medicine, law or engineering—work that nurtures our material life—can be called forms of 'external work', while activities such as journaling, therapy, mindfulness, yoga, art and writing—work that nurtures our inner life—is referred to as 'inner work'. Broadly, inner work encompasses the process of self-exploration, self-awareness and personal growth that people—whether they have experienced active traumatization (please refer to page 34 for an in-depth explanation of trauma) or not—engage in to better understand themselves and their emotions, thoughts, beliefs and behaviours.

It is a personal journey, and there is no one-size-fits-all approach. I believe every person can benefit from some amount of inner work in their life, because each one of us has been impacted by interpersonal and systemic trauma as part of living in a challenging world. There is no person who is 'above this' or who doesn't need inner work practice at some point. One has the freedom to choose a form of the practice that suits one's uniqueness.

I notice that when we urban Indians hear the word 'therapy', either we think of medical psychiatry, extreme forms of mental illness, psychiatric hospitals and the stigma attached to psychiatric medication, or we think of TV or film representations where an upset protagonist meets a misguided 'advice guru' masquerading as a counsellor and ends up being further harmed than helped. Some of us might even imagine dramatic, cathartic confessions happening inside a therapist's office, where every trauma pattern is instantly healed by the magician therapist in one 'breakthrough' session, after which the client is permanently 'cured' of their problem.

I name these ideas as 'therapy myths' in my work. What healing from trauma-based responses and patterns realistically looks like within our cultural context has not been written about very often. It is thus no surprise that our minds jump to such conclusions or extremes at the mere suggestion of accessing therapy. Even in 2024, there are few Indian TV shows that have done a good job of depicting therapy and healing for and by Indians.

### Inner work helps us understand why we believe something to be true

As a child, I heard many stories from my mother about what was culturally acceptable for girls to do when she was a teenager in

Mangalore. I remember our lively discussions about the differences between what her mother's culture taught her as 'good girl behaviour' and what she was passing onto me. The word 'culture' doesn't have one specific meaning. While it is powerful in shaping our minds, bodies and sexualities, it also moves and evolves over time. There are many types of cultures that impact us, and that impact is called 'conditioning'.

There is domestic culture (the norms in your home), religious culture (the norms of the religious group you or your family might belong to) and dating culture (social norms around relationships, including gender roles), among others. What therapists and researchers do know is that we are all products of many systems of psychological conditioning, and culture is one of those systems. Because psychological and social conditioning deeply impact the choices we make—whether we are consciously aware of it or not—I strive to make space for people's inner relationship with sexuality and culture to lead us to a deeper understanding of where they may be feeling stuck.

What our mothers, fathers, grandparents, cousins, schoolteachers, nannies, religious and spiritual gurus, priests and others tell us in our childhood about life gets interpreted by us, as children, as 'truth'. This is only natural. However, this is what creates this stubborn thing that's called 'psychological conditioning'. The movies and songs we consume contribute to it, as do the verbal and non-verbal strategies our families use to deal with life's many challenges.

All this impacts us first as children at home, then at school, then in college and workplaces and finally in the adult homes we ourselves go on to create. We often carry forward information from one life phase to the next without really stopping and asking how relevant that conditioning, that stored information, is for us. What was true for you at six, is it still true for you at thirty-six? Does that truth still hold meaning for the world around you?

## Inner work can bring awareness to 'internalized oppression'

Resmaa Menakem is one of my favourite writers. On colonial trauma, he writes that 'Oppressed people often internalize the trauma-based values and strategies of their oppressors'. This means that when people are traumatized by something for a very long period, they often lose connection with who they really are. They lose touch with who they were pre-trauma. They live in a state of ambiguity, low self-esteem and confusion, which is a state that is hard to maintain. So, to survive, they can take on the values of what their abusive oppressors hold true.

I have witnessed innumerable stories of internalized colonial mindsets leading to intense sex negativity in the inner lives of Indian people located all over the world. As Menakem says, very often traumatized or oppressed people are unaware of how deep this oppression lies within themselves. This is why it is called *internalized* oppression—the abuser's harmful ways of living have now become your own, and you don't even know it.

Inner work practices such as therapy, meditation, journaling, creating art and communal grief-sharing can lead us to a greater sense of agency around this internalized sense of oppression. It can empower us to separate beliefs around sex and sexuality that have been imposed upon us as normative, versus those that are indigenous to us.

## Inner work helps identify unprocessed trauma that we may not be able to see

Apart from cultural norms and norm-based oppression such as colonial trauma or religious trauma, which might repress what's natural and true for us as children or adults, it is essential to understand how broad the scope of trauma really is. So, what really is trauma? And why am I proposing that learning about it will help you have smoother, deeper and more intimate relationships?

For example, while having nightmares of your abusive ex every night can be traumatic, being fat-shamed everyday by your family can also be traumatizing. As research advances and society evolves, the definition of trauma also shifts and changes. Today, largely, we understand trauma not just as an individual event that caused some sort of harm to a person—such as an accident, an illness or the passing of a parent when one was a child (these are also very valid)—but also as an ongoing cause of distress in terms of deeply held harmful, unjust or misguided beliefs that lead people to shame, hurt, oppress, abuse or look down upon others. Examples include racism, sexism, misogyny, ableism and casteism, among others.

When trauma happens (no person escapes the knife of trauma in some way, shape or form)—when we get hurt, ill, violated, abused, pained, shamed, bullied or impacted by a lack of control over the events in our lives—our bodies adapt to that physical and emotional pain to keep us alive. If we were lucky as children, we had at least one secure adult around us who helped calm us and then repaired the hurt before it transformed into something more drastic.

A lot of us urban Indian adults had some form of stable, if not secure, adult to calm physical pain. Most Indian parents of any generation are extremely attentive to physical harm towards children. However, that same physically secure adult likely did not have the emotional tools to calm us down in the ways children need—at a more tender, heart-centred level (a concept that is explored in depth in Part 4 of this book). As the years went by, we never accessed any emotional repair or healing—and that adaptive pain became completely 'normal' to us.

Most people grow up with a curious mix of knowledge, values, judgements, pains, triggers, attitudes, behaviours, feelings and beliefs that come from the various people, places and events in our past. Without pausing to reflect on these, we may go through life never really understanding that underneath the surface of this carried-forward information lies an individual entity—a unique person with their own heart, mind, sexuality and spirit—who has the power to make their own choices, feel their own feelings, listen to their own mind and attune to their own body, gently and compassionately.

So, when we practise looking below the surface of someone's life story, we begin to understand more deeply how they're also uniquely shaped as sexual–emotional beings carrying their own unique mix of decades of stored information. We slowly start to recognize how living a mentally, sexually, emotionally, physically and spiritually well life is less about asking, 'What is wrong with me?', 'Who can fix me?' or 'What is the problem with you?', but more about reflecting on, 'What is that really happened to me?', 'How have I been impacted by it?' and, most importantly, 'How can I learn to live with it in a way that makes sense to me and that gives me clarity and power to lead my life as I want to?'

## Inner work can give us better coping skills for trauma

The understanding and insight that can come from truly finding answers to these essential questions over a long period of time can then help us make more empowered choices for the lives that we may really want to live. We then start to access the powerful, healing choice of keeping the harmful stories of our cultural conditioning aside, choosing the stories we want and making more considered choices within a larger society that might be slowly recovering from traumatization and disempowerment.

Please note that 'inner work' can involve various formal and informal techniques and practices of self-awareness. Every individual's and community's inner work process may unfold over time. Overall, therapists find that people engaging in inner work lead an enhanced quality of life, with greater self-acceptance, compassion, resilience and understanding.

## Therapy is a professional form of inner work

> 'Shame needs three things to grow exponentially in our lives: secrecy, silence and judgement.'
> —Dr Brené Brown

In my practice, I often meet people when a problem in their life has become acute and gotten out of hand. By the time most Indians choose to challenge the stereotypes against psychotherapy as a mental health practice, and take a courageous risk by entering offices like mine, more often than not something extreme has already happened. I meet highly functioning individuals whose partner drags them to a therapist as a last measure to save their marriage, and teenagers who are sent to therapy to be 'fixed' by their workaholic parents. I see new mothers who want to navigate postpartum depression, and young adults who are living together for the first time. I see newlyweds who want assistance with space sharing in inter-caste marriages, and queer people who are navigating aspects of their sexuality in an oppressive household culture.

I then have to work hard at explaining to these individuals, couples and families who are brave enough to seek professional support that therapy is not a magic pill—but is, at its core, a supportive long-term relationship that helps you see what you're not able to see in yourself. It is best to access therapy when the problems are not yet severe, and when life's circumstances are comfortable so that further problems can be nipped in the bud. Therapy is one of the best harm reduction practices possible.

Like any real relationship, it takes time for the establishment of trust. As you open up to the therapist of your choice about something challenging for you, the therapist's professional training is geared towards helping you find your own solutions to the challenges at hand. I like the metaphor of baggage and 'suitcases' to further understand the need for inner work and therapy.

As we may already know from the previous explanation of cultural conditioning, each human being is a complex mix of thoughts, feelings, sensations, behaviours, desires, hopes, values and more. Each relationship from childhood—or relational trauma (something negative that caused disruption in that relationship) at any stage of life—that one experiences leads one's psyche to gather more of these complexities. It is a natural process of psychological aging. Life's challenges tend to get more complex as we grow older. Many of these complexities that become part of our psychology live 'under the surface' of what's conscious to us, which is what we mean when we say something is 'subconscious'. So, while we may think we're uncomplicated and pattern-free, the truth is that nobody is truly so. Each person has their own inner world that is filled with its own complexities.

Now, if we don't take the time to organize these complexities for ourselves in some way, over time we end up with heavy, messy, chaotic baggage. We may feel like we want to be free and happy, but our chaos follows us wherever we go. We don't feel light, present or alive in our bodies; we feel burdened and blocked. However, when we do take the time to understand our inner chaos—which is the natural result of life's challenges—and put it in some form of order that makes sense to us, we end up with 'suitcases' instead.

With a system of organization, we can choose how many contents of our past we'd like to carry forward and how many we would like to leave behind. Some 'suitcases' are so heavy that their contents might never be fully organized—and that is also part of our human experience. Therapy often helps us discern the difference so that we can travel through life in the most liberated way possible.

## How to find a good-enough therapist for yourself

There are no 'perfect' therapists, partners, daughters, fathers, sons, mothers, trauma survivors, trauma perpetrators or therapy clients. There are only imperfect human beings who become 'good enough' for us over time and mutual effort. As a specialist in my field, I focus on working with three groups of Indian people: people who are looking to leave abusive relationships; people who have both survived and perpetrated sexual violence trauma; and people who are erotically marginalized (i.e., people whose sexualities are termed 'alternate' or different from the mainstream).

The root that connects the people I serve is traumatic distress, and the question I'm often trying to answer in my practice—'What's the most appropriate channel for the healing of this trauma for this particular individual in their own particular context?' Sometimes, it so happens that one person's lived experiences overlap all three groups, like some of the people whose lives I have talked about in this book. I've changed their real names and identities to protect their privacy, and they've given me their consent to share their stories of healing in therapy. I'm grateful for their courage to access professional support when they needed it and for their desire for others to benefit from their journey.

I often say on repeat in the therapy room—much to the chagrin of my clients—that time doesn't heal the wound; it often freezes it instead. We must heal it ourselves. We can't shame ourselves into healing—we need to approach our own wounds gently and with compassion. If some of these chapters motivate you to seek professional support for yourself, a family member or a friend, you should know that finding the right therapist is a process in itself. Psychotherapy and counselling include a vast array of practices, modalities, interventions and sensitivities. Some therapists embrace religion and spirituality within their practice, while others prefer not to. Some counsellors work with groups of people together, while others choose to limit their work to individuals and may have specific protocols about how they like to practise.

I am a depth-focused psychotherapist who uses art-based tools to form unique healing interventions for each of my clients. In my modality, sessions can run for 90 minutes, while other practitioners follow the traditional 45- to 60-minute therapy session format. Finding a therapist requires time, money and a desire to connect deeply with a trained person who shares values and worldviews with you. It is a process similar to dating, without the romantic or friendship angle. I'd suggest that some basic amount of trial and error is to be expected, and you may not find a match with the first or even the second professional.

## Relational therapists with creative approaches

Traditional psychotherapy prioritizes talking about the wounds while the body and its myriad languages take a backseat. In my formal and informal training in theatre, in art and then in trauma-informed art therapy itself, I learnt ways to bring the body's realities into the therapy room through art, music, poetry, drama and dance as well as through words. I learnt the language of somatics and found it mirrored in the ancient Indian science of yoga. I understood that especially for those of us of Indian origin—people who are just starting to name the impact of over a hundred years of colonial trauma—so many truths live outside of language. And so many truths have been passed on from one generation to the other in the form of stories and living history.

In a more relational style of therapy, you might find your therapist using the therapy relationship as a mirror for your patterns in relationships with people. You might gain insight into how you show up during power struggles or conflicts, or how you push people away without meaning to.

## Family therapists who work with groups of people together

There are so many common threads of sexual conflicts—familial conflicts around sexual values, sexual myths related to cultural taboos, relational complexities and sexual desires—that we Indians share as a people, even in our staggering diversity. I've seen that even simply *naming* the shared Indian relational–cultural realities that have been repressed from social consciousness due to their 'taboo nature' can lead to so much emotional freedom and powerful healing for so many of us.

One of the other major factors that keep us stuck in shame both as a society and as individuals is the very strict gaze of intergenerational conflict within our social systems. All of these are legitimate inner and outer realities and complexities that keep Indian families, couples and individuals stuck in layers of secrecy and codependency, which often lead to increased tension and relationship conflicts. It makes sharing space increasingly difficult.

When conflict isn't managed actively, it often becomes toxic. In popular psychology, when something is defined as toxic, it means it has become poisonous, which indicates it is dangerous to be around.

Over time, this toxicity can cause illness that then leads to more shame, distortion and stagnancy—which in turn leads to more ill-health. A family therapist is trained to help conventional and non-conventional family units to work through years of mismanaged relational conflict, to help members process traumatic family events such as deaths, accidents, illnesses, job losses and more and to help individuals gain greater awareness of trauma responses and how they impact each other.

## Traditional talk-based psychotherapists

Talk therapy isn't a space where you seek advice from a teacher or motivation from a life coach. This is an intellectual process that involves discussing thoughts, feelings and behaviours in a safe and supportive environment, which could then help you create changes in your life the way you'd like. There are many forms of talk therapy available to choose from, and if you're someone who prefers a primarily intellectual process, this might be a good pathway of healing and growth to look into.

Look for the following when you're seeking a therapist for sexual health challenges in the urban Indian setting:

- **Your therapist shouldn't make you feel judged for your sex life.**

  Look for someone who seems open to having a conversation with you about your decisions. If you still end up feeling judged, don't hesitate to bring it up to them and make your experience known. At its core, a successful therapy relationship requires both the therapist and the client to work on understanding each other.

- **Your therapist shouldn't guarantee healing outcomes or make promises to you about your health.**

  No therapist is supposed to promise you results. Therapy works when it is a good fit, when there is consent and when you're acting on the insights you're gaining from the process.

- **Your therapist must understand basic sexual health.**

  After a few sessions if you find that you're having to educate your therapist about sexual health and sexuality, then consider that their training may be outdated. If you're looking for support with challenges around alternative sexuality and more, this may not be a great fit.

Most professionals have a website with their qualifications and expertise listed publicly. Don't hesitate to ask them about this in the first session. Trust takes effort and time to establish. Please do remember that a therapist who works well for you may not work that well for your friend or family member because each of us is unique. Please do not force therapy on your close relationships.

## Chapter Takeaways

Inner work is the broad term for various processes of self-exploration, self-awareness and personal growth that people—whether they have experienced active traumatization or not—engage in to better understand themselves and their emotions, thoughts, beliefs and behaviours. It is a personal journey, and there is no one-size-fits-all approach.

Therapy is a professional form of inner work. While it is not a magic pill, with a trained professional, it can serve as a supportive long-term relationship that helps you see what you're not able to see in yourself. It is best to access therapy when the problems are not yet severe, and when life's circumstances are comfortable so that further problems can be nipped in the bud.

## Exercise 4: Questions to ponder over

Here are a few questions for you to think about as you complete this chapter. Think back to your environment growing up, as far back as you can. The further back you can go, the deeper your insights can be, as you move forward in the book.

• Growing up, what was your and your family's understanding of mental health? Was it easily discussed in your home? Was it treated as an open secret?

.........................................................................................................

.........................................................................................................

.........................................................................................................

.........................................................................................................

.........................................................................................................

.........................................................................................................

.........................................................................................................

.........................................................................................................

.........................................................................................................

.........................................................................................................

.........................................................................................................

- How were therapy or inner work practices viewed in your household?

.........................................................................................................

.........................................................................................................

.........................................................................................................

.........................................................................................................

.........................................................................................................

.........................................................................................................

.........................................................................................................

.........................................................................................................

.........................................................................................................

.........................................................................................................

- How did your family's views impact you?

.........................................................................................................

.........................................................................................................

.........................................................................................................

.........................................................................................................

.........................................................................................................

.........................................................................................................

.........................................................................................................

......................................................................................................

......................................................................................................

- What ideas, judgements, stereotypes or cultural stigmas do
  you carry today, about people who access therapy or those
  who take time out on a consistent basis to engage in inner
  work?

......................................................................................................

......................................................................................................

......................................................................................................

......................................................................................................

......................................................................................................

......................................................................................................

......................................................................................................

......................................................................................................

......................................................................................................

......................................................................................................

......................................................................................................

# CHAPTER 3

# 'I want to tell our son that I'm gay and that my wife knows.'

## *On coming out to the family as a sixty-year-old queer Indian man*

An Indian father's love isn't something that's easily translatable to words. Our urban Indian cultural mainstream is not a very verbose setting, unlike the white American TV sitcoms that so many of us have grown up watching. Even though young Indian people are increasingly seeking out the language for expressing emotional care and sorting out conflict, this is not really a society where we've been taught to sit at dinner tables and express, dissect or even process our innermost feelings for each other, especially when those feelings might be about our own biological family.

Familial love here is assumed, expected and required—and is demonstrated in non-verbal ways in most normative Indian families. Many generations of Indians accept this unspoken rule without challenge. It is considered common knowledge that you aren't supposed to question what is culturally assumed to be obviously given to you by your family. It is common to hear statements such as 'Of course your mother loves you—how can you even doubt that?

And why would she ever need to say it to you? You should already know it.' And if, for whatever reason, you do happen to question this assumption—especially if, unfortunately, you were born to a not very loving Indian mother or father—you should expect to be seen as the problem for even daring to want more. 'How dare you be so ungrateful?' is a very common statement in many Indian families. Let's look at it from the other side for a minute. Parenting in India, unlike its white-Western counterpart, is a socially approved twenty-five-year project. Culturally, Indian parents experience immense social ostracization and gossip, classism, caste-based oppression and more if their children don't turn out to be successful in socially approved ways. Here, parents don't expect that their children would move out of the family home at eighteen and then see them only once or twice a year. Nor is there an expectation that adult children would never take a loan from their families again. Instead, in India, parents—and in particular fathers—are expected to, and often do, express their love through a series of lifelong actions and cumulative acts of service for their children, even when they become legal adults.

While buying school textbooks and financing other expenses for children below the age of eighteen is a parental expectation common around the world, in India this often extends to fathers buying college textbooks, the child's first mobile phone and computer and perhaps even their first car. He may also file his children's first tax returns and manage their first investments and bank accounts. The responsibility extends to even finding suitable marriage partners.

These are some expected ways in which Indian fathers are expected to display love to their adult children. A statement like 'I love you and I'm here for you' is not commonly heard in this cultural context, simply because this is not a culture with a verbal orientation for emotional expression. Every culture has its normative 'love language'—the primary way one is comfortable receiving or giving love—and ours doesn't feature words of affirmation ... yet.

Many of us adult Indian 'children' are often starved of hearing the simple but loaded sentence: 'I love you, I'm proud of you and I'm here for you.' People are diverse in their needs, but more often than not adults like to hear expressions of vulnerability from their parents. 'Beta, I'm struggling. I'm sad that I won't be able to help you with money this month'—a statement that seems simple to one generation often creates anxiety, discomfort and shame for another generation.

So, when Mr J—who was tall, lean, Maharashtrian and almost sixty—filled his nearly hour-long first therapy session with a monologue about his son, Rohan, his sadness and their disconnection, I could tell that he was slightly different from the average Indian man. Rohan was all Mr J spoke about during our first several sessions—he described him as a sweet boy in need of rescuing, or rather, his father's help—despite me using all sorts of therapy tools to move his focus away from his son and towards himself.

I tried active listening, passive listening, imagery, confrontation, the dramaturgical 'empty chair' technique and even invited him to use some art tools as a way for him to go deeper beyond his surface-level narratives, but to no avail. It seemed like he wanted to do his best to convince me that he was a very doting father, and it was really Rohan, the struggling twenty-something son, that we needed to analyse. Mr J absolutely would not and could not talk about his own self in those first sessions.

Underneath Mr J's strict control of his therapy narrative, the anxiety was palatable. He came across as a strict but kind-hearted gentleman and had come into therapy expressing disappointment over the lack of connection he felt with his twenty-six-year-old son, who was studying in an engineering college in Maharashtra. Mr J said that he felt sad Rohan was away from home and that he missed him.

This wasn't my typical distressed parent complaining about their son's life choices. Even under severe mental distress, rarely do Indian parents of Mr J's generation show up for therapy on their own—and that too with a queer Indian woman much younger than them. Something was unique about him, and I had to allow him to retain control until he felt safe enough to relax in my presence.

At his eleventh therapy session, I placed a handheld mirror in front of Mr J and said, 'Please look at your face in this mirror when you say your son's name.'

He looked shocked and said, 'Huh?'

I repeated, 'Look at your face in this mirror when you say your son's name. What do you see? Tell me.'

'Umm … I don't know … I just see my face.'

'Say your son's name slowly, please.'

Mr J mouthed 'Rohan' in the mirror. There was an awkward silence between us for a moment.

'So, Rohan feels sad that his father is so far away from him,' said Mr J, shifting to verbal processing. 'And I need to tell Rohan that …' The shock of looking at himself had been distressing.

'J, let's relax into this silence that is hanging between us. Please close your eyes with me and imagine your son's face right now in your mind.'

I gave him a minute to settle in. He seemed uncomfortable yet eager to take my instruction. 'When you open your eyes, look at your face in the mirror and tell me exactly what you see. Don't worry about being right or wrong—just observe.'

Eventually, he said, 'I see a person who looks just like Rohan, but not as young, not as agile, not as … honest.'

'Honest?'

'Yes, honest. I have not been honest.' Mr J slowly looked away from his own mirror image and stared at me with a deadpan expression. We spent the next fifteen minutes in a comfortable, almost meditative quietude. He knew that I was waiting for him to share more about what he had just revealed. It was the first thing he had chosen to share about himself in eleven therapy sessions. My pauses helped affirm to him that he was still in control. I would not force him to tell me what was waiting to be told.

'I am a gay man,' he finally said. 'I have a wife, I have a son, and I am a disappointment to them both. I had been dishonest with Ratna, my wife, for many, many years, but right from our wedding day, she knew that I was not fully interested in her. I was always a bright student and studied at the top engineering and management institutes of the country. Even though my father encouraged me to study, I had a big responsibility to provide for my family, because we did not come from money. Ratna is the one who pushed me to see a counsellor, because she knew. I have never said this out loud to anyone but her and my sister: I am gay. I am gay. I am gay. It is Rohan who does not deserve this.'

'What does Rohan not deserve, J?'

'A sick baba like me.'

The session ended abruptly there. He left with a quick nod. I wondered if he would return to therapy.

Like every therapist, I believe that healing is inherently painful, but starting one's healing journey without addressing the wound is often more traumatizing over time. Sometimes what surfaces in therapy with a safe, trusted and liked professional is so intense that the light is too blinding, and people retreat into the darkness. It is safer there, in the second identity that us queer people create to keep us accepted by wider society.

We are more accepted in India if we don't reveal these truths about ourselves. We are taught that our truths are 'selfish desires' that can be avoided. We are sent to conversion therapy where a homophobic 'clinical expert' tries to talks us out of feelings for people with the same gender or sexual identity. In extreme cases, our parents and worried family members are convinced by the same experts that our nerves need to be shocked to change our brain's wiring—and we are electrocuted. This is not fiction, dear reader. These are the punishments that queer people have received for coming out, and all of this has been in the news. Why would we trust the therapist community?

Mr J's journey was unique, though. And he did come back. Over the next few months, he became even more eager for regular therapy, asking for appointments more than once a week. He started to express feelings of deeper trust in me. Still, I wondered, besides clinical skill, what drew this elderly queer person towards me? What made him stay?

Over time, he revealed that he had seen my website once through social media, and that the boldness he'd sensed in me reminded him of his sister, Supriya. She was in her forties and worked as a professor of mathematics in Chennai. Twenty years ago, she had chosen to not marry at a time when such choices were even more frowned upon in South India.

Supriya was the one who Mr J had confided in when he had first experienced adolescent love towards a boy in school. He had then secretly dated a sports coach named Sujay for five years before succumbing to familial pressure and marrying Ratna. Supriya would often host Sujay and Mr J in her home, where they would spend hours watching Tamil cinema over hot chips and tea. The relationship ended the night Mr J received news that he had graduated B-school—he abruptly asked Sujay to leave Supriya's house and told him to never call again.

Mr J had already agreed to marry Ratna and believed that 'everything would be fine and normal' after marriage. After all, wasn't his sexual orientation just a perversion? What would his friends and family say if he did not marry a woman, especially after graduating from the country's top B-school? The choicest Marathi slurs for his 'type' of people came to his mind.

We queer people experience an incredible kind of aloneness. In a community-driven culture like India, this aloneness is like being parched swimming in an ocean—there's water everywhere but you can't drink it as you're not a fish. If you happen to be a queer person who also succeeds academically or at work in India, the internal isolation you might feel is magnified. You might even start to believe the second identity you've built to pass as an 'excellent civilian'.

Mr J was experiencing intense feelings of shame for living his truth. He was raised in an environment where his truth was unnatural and impure—it was a perversion and an assault to his manhood and to his family's reputation. He then learnt to create a hidden self inside while presenting himself as 'normal' on the outside.

Mr J and I spent three years in a strong therapeutic alliance. He stayed in individual therapy for a hectic year, during which he processed a lot of his own internalized shame about being gay. We practised speaking small doses of authentic truth, which he then practised at home with his wife. We then shifted to regular couples' therapy where Ratna and Mr J worked on breaking up with intention, with the least harm possible to each other. It was during this process and under the kind, compassionate gaze of his wife— who was leaning into working her way out of this marriage and supporting her husband's truth—that Mr J truly began to become fully vulnerable.

The two of them would keep a couples' therapy journal in which they would write to each other every week. I would serve as a gentle witness, melting walls when they came up and teaching the couple to create new boundaries where necessary. This was a couple that had a solid foundation of friendship, so between the three of us there was a beautiful, inviting and warm energy. Therapy became a nurturing cocoon for the changes that were taking place. They were able to retain their friendship after the rough parts that any breakup brings.

In his third year of inner work, Mr J decided to stop trying to control his son. He learnt that hiding important information and essential realities about oneself from the very people one cares about is a way of subtly sabotaging those very relationships and keeping genuine love at bay. This form of covert manipulation is something we Indians are taught to do from childhood so as to not rock the boat too much in a people-pleasing culture. Mr J managed to unlearn it. By the end of the third year, feeling more in-tune with his body, his mind, his heart and his spiritual truth, he was able to have the honest conversation about his sexuality that he had been wanting to have with his son for the last decade.

Rohan was not surprised at all. In fact, he had suspected all along that his father was queer. He was concerned for his mother, as he thought her feelings had not been centred in this process. However, she assured him that the reason she had chosen to stay with his father this long was because they were friends first, and she wanted him to get the support he needed. They all took time off from inner work as a family to nurture their grief, both as a unit and individually, as people breaking away from inauthenticity and oppression.

Over the course of these three intense years of trauma work, Mr J projected many hats onto me, of which I wore all those that fit me within the boundaries of our alliance. I played the metaphoric sister, friend, confidante, daughter, wife, gentle nurturer, truth-telling mirror, bullshit-free life coach and somatic healer to him. He told me that he kept coming back to therapy even when he felt like melting into his shame because there were parts of him that had never been shown to another person but which had felt understood and even mirrored when he talked to me. This was because of my own identity as an Indian queer person.

He said that practising while staying in the light of truth-telling despite judgement and pushback felt so good to him that he was able to take gentle steps with the support of his family towards living openly as a gay elder in his community of close confidants and friends. Of course, since we still have a long way to go before our country is a safe space for queer people, Mr J keeps his sexuality hidden at his post-retirement job at a nonprofit organization. For now, he is thrilled to be able to live with self-leadership between trusted friends and family members. However, he does wish for a safer, less harm-filled future for others with a truth like his, and a less traumatic journey for the family members of queer Indians.

*'J's loneliness lived unexpressed; he seemed like a weary traveller living a double life, alien to his own self. Words mask his grief as Ratna waits for her old friend to return to her from inside her husband's dead frame.'*

Notes to myself in my art therapy journal after a session with Ratna and Mr J.

## Chapter Takeaways

Practicing emotional honesty in a society, which encourages secrecy, shame and living a double life for fear of what others will say, is a tremendous challenge. Family-oriented Indians, who identify as queer and are not part of the online generation, are at the forefront of this challenge, risking social ostracization for speaking their truth with little support. While intergenerational bonds are complex to navigate as is, living an unashamed, healthy life as a queer individual in a society steeping with unaddressed sexual shame, adds additional relational burdens. Indian family systems require a lot more legal, social and systemic support than is currently available to ensure their long-term well-being.

## Exercise 5: Understand the stages of queer identity formation

A large part of growing up in the Indian cultural context is to learn how to 'adjust'. From childhood, the narrative we are taught is that life is not an entirely individual journey. It is a collective, family-oriented journey where it is important to learn to live with different personality types. We're taught to avoid speaking directly about what we need, especially with the elders in our family, since our needs might inconvenience them or cause them emotional pain.

While this cultural expectation teaches us the value of compromise, this can very often also lead to people not being able to ask for what they might really need to live a healthy life. Living dual lives—one for our families, where we perform roles to meet sociocultural expectations; and one for ourselves, where we permit ourselves to live authentically according to our true needs, desires, wants, values and expectations—is a pervasive experience for so many Indians.

Mr J's case example shows us the challenges of living in fragments, and what the psychosomatic cost of that duplicity is for so many of us. As a queer Indian man, Mr J struggled with his gay identity throughout his marriage. His wife, being aware of his sexual identity, wanted to support him to live in his truth, but they were afraid of being judged by their son, their friends and extended family and the larger spiritual and religious community that they belonged to.

It is a topic on which our country has heated value-conflicts. It is strange to think that a subject so essential and primary as one's gender and sexual orientation—an area of life that directly impacts health and well-being—is rarely broached by Indian families. This chapter explored the connections between intergenerational roles in Indian families, the cycle of sexual shame and the realities of living an alternate sexual identity in a culture that is very slowly trying to broaden what it accepts as 'normal'.

As an extension of reading this chapter, I invite you to think about the long-drawn process of 'coming out' for queer people living in non-accepting or less-accepting cultures where attacks, insults and mockery await them at every turn. We hear of 'coming out' on social media and of TV shows on which queer characters share their struggles and celebrations. But what, really, does this term mean?

## Let's explore

'**Coming Out**' is an ongoing and dynamic process whereby LGBTQ+ individuals discover, acknowledge and choose to disclose their sexual orientation and/or gender identity to themselves and others. Coming out is not a one-time process. Queer individuals living in societies where queerness is either punishable legally—or socially through norms and rules—often have to declare their truths repeatedly, facing the risks of social isolation or even attacks and harm each time.

There are six known stages of the 'coming out' process according to clinical psychologist and sex therapist, Dr Vivienne Cass, who in 1979, developed one the first theories of modern LGBT QIA+ identity development which normalized queerness in a heteronormative society instead of treating homosexuality and bisexuality themselves as a problem to be studied.

The stages are:

**Identity Confusion:** I am 'not normal' when compared to my larger culture or peers.

**Identity Comparison:** Yes, I may have attractions and feelings, but I am not ready to label myself within a non-heteronormative identity.

**Identity Tolerance:** I'm beginning to be okay with some parts of this identity and am starting to want or have more queer friends.

**Identity Acceptance:** I'm able to have a more self-accepting view of my sexuality.

**Identity Pride:** I'm learning about queer subcultures, but I might also be having a lot of 'us versus them' feelings and experiencing resentment and anger towards mainstream society.

**Identity Synthesis:** I'm more able to accept that there may be trustworthy allies in heterosexual communities and the 'us versus them' dichotomy isn't entirely accurate.

I use this model in therapy to help queer folks organize both their struggles and joys of queer identity formation and maturation. Many queer folks share feelings of relief, similar to how I felt when I first applied this model to my own queerness. Others find this model limiting and alienating to their individual expectations, and that is worked through and accepted in therapy as well.

No theory of lived experience can fit all sizes and shapes of experiences, however I must emphasize that organizing and studying a natural part of human existence that has been demonized and shamed for centuries, is to be celebrated as a massive step of a collective de-shaming process of healing.

While Mr J had the financial and educational privilege to be able to access and afford therapy, some queer Indian people may never choose to come out to their families. They may risk living with covert (hidden) or even overt (more obvious) depression, loneliness and social alienation and with feelings of disconnection and emotional numbness. They may even consider self-harm and suicide.

Subcultures of queer communities have been thriving in the margins in India since time immemorial. Indian people misinformed by a massive colonial hangover declare that queerness is a 'Western concept', but queerness has always been an integral part of Indian society. 'Temple sculptures from Konark and Khajuraho to the Kamasutra and other ancient literary materials contain enough references to evidence that ancient India accommodated a whole range of sexual behaviours', writes scholar R.K. Dasgupta in his 2011 article, 'Queer sexuality: a cultural narrative of India's historical archive'. Ruth Vanita's book, *Love's Rite* is another fantastic document of non-English-speaking young couples all over India who fought for the right to marry and live together, outside of ideological movements and state and religious sanction. Vanita says that many such couples did not use any identity whatsoever to concretize their relationship. They did not use the words queer, or lesbian, gay, transgender, or even homosexual, because they were not trying to define an individual identity; they were trying to define a relationship. In doing so, she names the difference between modern,

Western culture and non-Westernized Indian culture. She says, 'the former is often (not always) focused on individual identity while the latter on relationships within which identities form themselves in relation to others'.

Over the last ten to fifteen years, India has seen a lot of legal, social and psychological shifts on this topic. I remember sitting in a queer support group meeting in Delhi in 2009 with a friend who had been seeing a psychiatrist for conversion therapy in Kerala. He had been forced to go for conversion therapy by his parents, who threatened to stop allowing him to stay with them and even to disown him. Therapists, doctors and counsellors at the time did not have access to training in queer-affirmative mental, physical and sexual health support in their course education nor was there an expectation for them to get this training. Social media information also did not exist as it does today.

At the time, since homosexuality was still considered illegal, our support group meetings could do little more than offer ourselves as 'safe-enough' people, along with some temporary housing support on our own ragged couches for distressed queer people threatened with harm and abandoned by their own families.

*'History owes an apology to these people and their families. Homosexuality is part of human sexuality. They have the right to dignity and to be free of discrimination. Consensual sexual acts of adults are allowed for the LGBT(QIA) community.'*

*—Justice Indu Malhotra, retired judge and senior counsel of the Supreme Court of India.*

Legal rights for the queer community and the different identities that come under that large umbrella are in a better place now than they were even ten years ago. Delhi, Mumbai, Bangalore, Chennai and Kolkata today have created formal and informal public queer organizations, support groups, listening circles and safe spaces for coming out. There are parent support groups even in smaller cities such as Nagpur, Coimbatore, Kochi and Visakhapatnam.

I have been introduced to thriving subcultures of queer communities that exist all by themselves, organized by the members in their own homes or in quiet restaurants and street corners. It is nothing but resilience that helps oppressed communities when social acceptance is so traumatic. When communities are told to keep out of the public eye, they do not just stop existing—rather, they find ways to exist despite the oppression, even risking harm and abuse from those who do not understand, because human truths cannot just be deleted from existence.

## Exercise 6: *Create an inner work journal*

Earlier, I'd suggested keeping a journal as you travel through this book. Journal writing is popularly known as expressive writing. It is an act of writing to yourself freely, with abandon, without censorship. Therapists and researchers have found that it helps to psychologically reduce levels of anxiety, grief and stress. It provides an inexpensive and always accessible channel for intense feelings and unanswered questions by allowing the writer to find meaning in whatever is being expressed in the act of journaling.

Journal writing prompts given in this book have been carefully designed for you to explore these themes deeply and find resonance in your own life. You could add your own creative edge to your journal by making art or adding your favourite scent to its pages. You could also purchase one that can be locked for greater privacy.

*Here are a few journal prompts for you to consider, especially if you are a friend, family member or relative of someone who identifies as queer:*

- Do you know Indian queer people in your own life? Who are they? How do you experience their lives?

  Yes ☐    No ☐

- Do you find that you're a 'safe-enough' person for them to trust you? What could you do further to make yourself a safe-enough person to be trusted by someone whose gender and sexual orientation might be different from yours?

  Yes ☐    No ☐

- What are some stereotypes, biases, insults or shame-inducing lies you may have heard about gay, lesbian, bisexual or transgender people? How did you try to subvert them?

....................................................................................................

....................................................................................................

....................................................................................................

....................................................................................................

....................................................................................................

....................................................................................................

....................................................................................................

....................................................................................................

....................................................................................................

....................................................................................................

..........................................................................................................

..........................................................................................................

..........................................................................................................

..........................................................................................................

..........................................................................................................

• Can you think of ways in which Ratna and Rohan from the narrative above could be supported better in their own lives? If this was a family close to you and they trusted you as a close friend who knew of their struggles, how would you try and support them?

..........................................................................................................

..........................................................................................................

..........................................................................................................

..........................................................................................................

..........................................................................................................

..........................................................................................................

..........................................................................................................

..........................................................................................................

..........................................................................................................

..........................................................................................................

..........................................................................................................

..........................................................................................................

.................................................................................................................................

.................................................................................................................................

.................................................................................................................................

.................................................................................................................................

.................................................................................................................................

Families and friends of queer people who stand up and advocate for queer rights despite living under systems of oppression also suffer immense isolation, attack, physical and emotional harm and shaming behaviour from some members of mainstream society. There is a term for the type of trauma we experience indirectly when someone close to us is harmed. It's called secondary trauma. Secondary trauma can be a difficult experience to understand, especially when the person undergoing primary trauma struggles to get their needs for repair, justice, accountability and even soothing met.

# CHAPTER 4

# 'We've stopped having sex and we don't know why.'

## *On wanting to be more sexually connected, but not knowing where to begin again*

Have you ever been bitten by a leech? They're bloodsucking parasites found in moist environments. They attach themselves to the skin of their hosts, causing enough harm to feel a sting but not enough harm to need medical attention. I find leeches to be similar to this entity called shame that lives in our inner world, in our inner environment. Just like shame, leeches can be painful, draining and hard to detach from—yet, you often can't tell when you're bitten by one. Most people do not know that their lives are being quietly drained by shame.

Bindu and Rajeev lived in a quiet neighbourhood in Baroda. She liked to sing as a hobby, he liked to paint. Rajeev's father had been a retired government officer until he passed away a few years ago. His mother, Ninaben, was a Gujarati schoolteacher and self-taught playwright who now lived by herself. Bindu and Rajeev lived next door. This was a family that had a shared love for creative expression and, to the outside eye, their personalities were well-matched.

With conjoined apartments, each subunit had space to follow their own rhythms while being close to each other. With so much privilege as well as having shared hobbies and interests, one would typically expect things in this family to have remained calm and 'good' for long periods of time. Alas, if only textbook ideas of marriage and life were always true! The reality was that Bindu and Rajeev were in an inter-caste marriage. They had challenged many social norms to create a life together. Unfortunately, it led to Bindu becoming estranged from her parents, who had been against their union due to caste-based judgements about Rajeev. Although Bindu's family considered themselves socially progressive and open-minded, in matters of marriage caste played an important role.

Both Bindu and Rajeev were architects by profession. They had met in college, were devoted to their careers and did not want biological children. They had both helped their families financially as they had not been well-off growing up. Ninaben had almost adopted Bindu as her own daughter after Bindu's own family turned hostile. So, what happened for this couple to access therapy? What went 'wrong', you might ask? Isn't therapy only for couples who are on the verge of breakdown? Shouldn't their shared values, love and kindness for each other and an accepting mother-in-law automatically have led to a beautiful life together?

Urban Indian socialization tells us that inner work must be sought only when crisis hits. It looks down upon therapy overall, and specifically couples' therapy is seen as a highly pathologized experience in which a doctor or an advice guru lectures you endlessly on how to fix your problems and stay together regardless of what happens between the partners. The urban Indian TV representations of mental health professionals are often inaccurate and even insulting to the reality of what happens inside of therapy.

Like most therapists, I love facilitating people towards new choices that break old patterns. Couples' therapy is a specific clinical skill that requires advanced study and an internship during which a therapist is trained to create space for couples and families of all types to deepen their understanding of themselves together in various ways. This space can transform a couple's and family's life experiences through learning to become more vulnerable with each other, learning to offer empathy and compassion when stuck in blame and judgement, practicing accountability for harm caused in relationships, learning each other's trauma history to serve each other better and understanding the deeper wisdom behind each other's conflict styles.

The goal of couples and family therapy is not always to stay together. For some people there is tremendous power in realizing that they truly do not want to be together. Therapy can help make those realizations conscious. I teach Indian couples and families to learn to break up more consciously if that is what they choose, to ask for time apart with intention, to create more structure around privacy and consent in shared domestic spaces and to accept and engage with each other's sexual truths in a more relational way.

Rajeev was a growth-oriented person with good experiences with therapy during his college days. He was aware that there is more to romance, sex, marriage or long-term relationships than meets the eye. Without understanding how trauma naturally shows up in our adult relationships—especially the safe, secure, long-term ones— and how to address it, Rajeev knew that we can quickly become dejected by our own fantasies about how easy and nice a good relationship 'should' be. The romantic movies we watch leave us with the message that if you find the right person, everything will just naturally flow. Nothing could be further from the truth.

So, it was Rajeev who contacted me first, asking for a family therapy session with his wife and his mother also in attendance. He said he only wanted one session during which he could use my couple therapy skills to explain to Bindu and Ninaben that they were both being, in his words, 'overdramatic'. He said that although the first two years of his marriage had passed in jubilant celebration and an easy, natural flow of being together, there had been a lot of conflict lately. He was suddenly feeling as if he was being pulled in opposite directions by his mom and his wife. He labelled himself as 'helplessly stuck in the middle'. From being a harmonious family, they were slowly becoming fragmented.

Although he knew it had something to do with trauma, Rajeev wanted help to go deeper. While he was able to trust Bindu and himself to navigate everyday marital conflict together, he was getting frustrated that he had completely lost desire for sex—and, in some ways, for Bindu, whom he still loved deeply. Bindu, being the partner with the higher libido in the relationship, needed sex and physical touch for connection. Touch was her primary love language, but the more she asked for it in the ways that she did, the more resistant Rajeev became to her demands. And the more resistant he became, the louder, angrier and more intense Bindu's feelings of rejection and abandonment would get.

This spiral would push Rajeev to go to his mother's house next door to distract himself. He would help Ninaben with domestic chores and wait for Bindu to calm down. This behaviour would make Bindu feel even more abandoned because she thought her partner had left her when things were difficult and there was no one there to soothe her pain. The expectation to hold Bindu's intense feelings would make Rajeev more hostile.

However, while at his mother's house, Rajeev had to hear her constantly bring up stories of his father.

Ninaben would confess that she felt that had he been alive, she would probably have been better off. They would have been living in a better apartment, in a busier neighbourhood, in a larger city with a more secure financial provider. She would then nudge Rajeev to have children so that her own life could have more meaning and security. Rajeev would resist this pressure too, he would experience a 'shutting down' and experience immense frustration.

When Rajeev went back to his own apartment, he would find Bindu curled up in bed, crying. They would fall asleep without discussing their argument further. This would happen at least once a week. Rajeev expressed feeling like a terrible partner and wanting to run away from all of this. He could not believe that this was the same family system that over a year ago was living in almost perfect harmony. It had been one year since Bindu and Rajeev had found themselves in this cycle, and also one year since they last had sex. The tension in the room was so thick you could cut it with a knife.

It was a bustling Thursday afternoon six weeks into our therapeutic alliance, and there was enough mutuality and comfort in the room to teach this couple to start digging under their surface-level feelings. I thanked Rajeev for sharing deeply in the first session and validated his understanding of looking below the surface that he brought into the room with him. Looking at his stooped shoulders, I asked, 'Rajeev, how do you support your wife when she is angry with you?' Bindu, an introverted, energetic woman in her early thirties, angrily looked on.

Bindu had earlier finished narrating her experience of feeling like her beloved husband didn't want her. She had taken up thirty minutes of session time, breaking down multiple times, to frame questions such as 'What has changed? Why don't you want me anymore? Can you tell me what I can do better? What do you need from me?'

Rajeev had a more detached, observant demeanour about him. Each time Bindu asked him why, he seemed to physically retreat from her question. His shoulders would drop, his chest would deflate and he would quietly roll his eyes and look towards me.

When I asked him how he supported his wife when she was angry with him, he looked visibly confused.

'Support her when she is angry? What does that mean?'

'People in healthy adult relationships support each other not only when they're feeling positive about each other, but also when they're experiencing something seemingly negative. Are there ways in which you can contain your wife's anger, even if it is directed towards you and you do not want it?'

Rajeev became pensive.

There was a long silence, so Bindu started to offer her perspective.

'Well, he always buys me ice-cream the next day and he always calls before important presentations and—'

'Bindu, can we allow Rajeev to take his time to come up with an answer?' I interrupted. 'When you swoop in and relieve his anxiety of not knowing his answer, you're actually taking on two roles in your relationship—you're doing something we call "over-functioning".'

'Okay, what should I do though?' she asked hesitatingly. 'He's not a bad guy, he just shuts down—'

'And then you try and force him open. How has that worked for you?'

Bindu looked shocked.

'When you over-function, Bindu, have you considered that it could be a way for you to relieve your own anxiety?' I said. 'When we are stressed, we tend to go back to childhood ways of managing stress and conflict. Most people don't learn to make these internalized behaviours more conscious and go on repeating patterns. A repeated pattern then becomes a habit, and it takes time to unlearn bad habits. So, try waiting for Rajeev. Look at the impact your words have on his body. Your anger is powerful—trust it.'

This seemed to help Rajeev take up more space in the session. It seemed to make him feel more understood. He finally said, 'I think I understand what you mean by supporting Bindu when she is angry with me. No, I don't actually do that. I tend to want to leave.'

'What do you feel when she is angry with you?'

'I feel ashamed.'

'Okay, hold that feeling as it is surfacing right now. Tune into it. Why do you feel ashamed when your wife feels abandoned by you, do you know?'

Bindu's eyes sparkled as her husband's vulnerability entered the room. This time, she raised her hand for permission to speak, but I asked her to wait and let him unfold without interruption.

Our attachment styles are gateways to understanding why we communicate in specific ways in intimate relationships. All human beings relate to each other through something called 'attachment'. According to attachment therapist Dr Stan Tatkin, people's attachment can be island-like, wave-like or anchor-like. Sometimes, anxiously attached people (waves) can unintentionally take up a lot of the space in the relationship. In their bid for emotional connection, they can ask for the same thing repeatedly and think that they're helping their partner understand them better.

However, if they're paired with someone who takes longer to process their feelings and who remains a little distant from their own intensity (islands), then the anxiously attached partner's style of communication can shut the distant partner down. For the more emotionally distant partners, this experience of passionate intensity from their partners can feel overwhelming.

Bindu quickly adjusted her pace and waited eagerly for more of his truth. Her ability to do so demonstrated how much she wanted Rajeev to understand her, and how open she was to learn how to help him do that. 'When she gets angry with me and cries, I feel that I have failed the one job I am supposed to perform in a marriage,' said Rajeev eventually. 'I should feel attracted to her every day and I should want to sleep with her every night. I should make her feel like her body is the most beautiful and that she is the most desired woman on this planet. I should take care of her, especially since she left her parents to be with me—and because we fought against society to hold our own. So, when I don't do any of this, or I'm not able to, I feel that maybe she is better off without me. I am failing her.' One could feel the weight of all that Rajeev was expressing that afternoon. It felt burdensome. 'Rajeev, do you know that I too feel like a failure when you don't sleep with me?' sighed Bindu.

One of the ways in which our cultural conditioning harms us is that it holds an unrealistic view of dating and marriage. Despite having religious and moral stances against breakup or divorce, our culture doesn't actually teach us how to first survive and then thrive with someone long-term. During childhood, many of us Indians are discouraged from spending too much time with people of gender identities that aren't our own. After puberty, boys and girls are taught that dating will distract from studies, and that it is only something one should do when one is serious enough to get married.

While the cultural wisdom here, as I take it, is to perhaps become a whole person before getting attached to someone, this message gets implemented as an extreme form of policing of relationships among young people. Even schools actively discourage and sometimes punish the formation of young couples. This has led to the creation of a culture as it stands today—one full of young people with poor dating skills and abilities, low awareness of the challenges of other gender identities and very unrealistic expectations of what happens after you attach yourself to someone you like.

Once you're of age, most Indians are then pushed into marriage by their families, which is a lifelong commitment. So, basically, people are walking into a difficult life challenge that has the potential to make or break one's well-being with next to no knowledge or preparation. Relationships, like all arenas of life, come with their own learning curve. Some of us learn quickly and adapt, while others may need more support depending on who we are and what happened to us before we came into that relationship. Expecting one's long-term romantic experience to be 'naturally easy' because one's partner is 'the right one for me' speaks of little awareness of the reality of commitment.

As Dr Tatkin says, 'Everyone is a burden up close. There is no person who is low maintenance in an intimate relationship.' And this is because human beings come with complicated nervous systems filled with unmet needs, desires, longings and wishes. Our bodies are systems of information that are responding to each moment in their own unique way. This is why you may have a different reaction from others to the same situation.

In an intimate relationship, we have to learn to hold space for the feelings, triggers and experiences of both participants. What we're not taught is that one of the functions of a 'safe-enough' relationship is to create space for each partner to be able to confront what's buried under the surface for them so that they can choose their habits, reactions and responses consciously and live a wiser life. And relationship conflict is one of the only ways that we realize that something may be brewing underneath.

# Being in an adult relationship means you're going to have to learn to deal with conflict like an adult

Do you remember watching your parents repair fights at the family dinner table? Do you have a memory of your father approaching your mother in front of you, naming his triggers that led him to raise his voice and then him making space to listen to your mother's anger and hurt feelings? If you do, you're part of the exception. This would be an example of healthy repair after a relationship conflict. Most urban Indians that I talk to and meet, my friends, my extended family members or other Indian therapists I consult with have not seen relationship repair, either at home or on TV. There are no examples for ordinary people to even know what it takes to genuinely apologize to one's partner, to ask for forgiveness, to bid for sexual connection or to transform painful emotions into relationship wisdom.

As young adults, we are implicitly taught these two ideas, of which most of us choose one as a conscious or subconscious belief:

- Find the 'right person' and then life will be easy. The right person will love you for all your flaws and not make you uncomfortable in any way.

- Settle down with anyone who has some similar interests to you and keep putting in the work. Even if your partner doesn't put in the work with you, take whatever little love you get because no relationship should be abandoned. Divorce and breakups are shameful and bad.

The reality, though, is more in the middle, and hence more complex. There is no formulaic 'right person' created for you to match with and who complements you perfectly. There are only 'right relationships', in which the dynamics that partners create with each other enhance a state of ease, play, understanding and intimacy together.

These dynamics come after making good-enough (not perfect— no one is perfect) attempts to lean towards each other despite disliking some parts of the other or even being turned off by a few characteristics of the relationship. The moment one of the partners takes the relationship for granted, gives up on themselves, runs away from their triggers or places external blame for all things hard, the quality of the relationship suffers.

Over the next several months, Bindu and Rajeev learnt a form of this in their therapy journey. They learnt that over time, like many couples, they had started to take each other's needs for granted. Rajeev expected Bindu to have less intense feelings because her sorrow would make him feel like he was failing. Bindu expected Rajeev to want to prioritize time and desire for her, but she was asking in a harsh, scolding way without revealing her own feelings of rejection. Each of them was playing a part in the dysfunctional cycle that, at the time, was dominating their relationship and blocking them from deepening their understanding of each other.

The most uplifting part about working with this couple was that they held themselves accountable to what they said they wanted. They each did their part. This is a key ingredient to successful conflict healing and repair. Each week, I felt honoured to witness their energy in practicing deeper listening. They caught their shame spirals faster and set time apart weekly to discuss their innermost feelings and insights with each other. Over time, Bindu's feelings of intense abandonment lessened as she turned inwards and began to 'sit with' her needs more deeply instead of instantly expecting Rajeev to hold them all for her. This gave Rajeev more space to receive his wife's desires more completely.

Rajeev practised breaking the cycle of using his mother's chores as a distraction from his shame. He also learnt to address his feelings as they surfaced in conflict with Bindu and stopped trying to escape them. He put in place a 'time-out' system for himself and left the bedroom when Bindu's demands triggered him. As they had created mutual trust by then, she trusted him to come back to her more actively after he was feeling more open. This helped him feel less attacked, which opened his heart and his body more to making love with Bindu.

Triggers never go away, and we should stop expecting them to. Like our feelings, triggers are part of the language system of the body. They are your nervous system's way of telling you what your deepest needs are. The only thing we can do about our triggers is to understand them and build a relationship with them. This changes our perspective towards what we perceive to be problems in ourselves that we need to erase.

Changing our perspective deepens our hearts and brings compassion towards ourselves and our partners. In healthy and safe relationships, both people get to this understanding with intention, effort and time. In abusive relationships, triggers escalate into harm, feelings become attacks and partners aren't able to transform their shame spirals. Thus, chronic hurt and harm ensue.

It's also important to remember that sex and togetherness ebb and flow even between the healthiest of couples. This is normal. People in the most loving and conscious relationships get bored of each other some days; they fantasize about sex with strangers even while they are in true love with each other. Numerous changes happen in the body over time. Our bodies increase and decrease in size depending on our life circumstances, our skin stretches and stretch marks appear, moles sprout and our features shift over time. This is natural. Even orgasms become stronger or weaker as the body moves through illness, accidents, childbirth, childrearing and other life events.

Experiencing any of these changes in yourself in your loved ones does not mean that you're automatically 'out of love'. Experiencing repeated conflicts does not indicate that you have outgrown the love you have for your partner, as popular media makes us believe. It could mean that the time has come for your relationship to deepen and move to its next natural stage of maturity, provided everyone involved is committed to growth.

When people ask me why I write so much about all aspects of life and wellness when my therapy work focuses on sex and sexuality, I tell them it's because I see human sexuality as a part of attachment and relationship. I don't view sexuality as an isolated part of life with no connection to anything else. Among the younger generations of Indians who have more access to dating and greater permission to explore sexuality than the older generations, there is a common confusion between sexual chemistry and good sex. People often conflate the two and think these will bring the same results. However, these are not the same.

Often when we feel 'good chemistry' with someone, we jump to the conclusion that since the two of us are really attracted to each other, the act of sex with that person will also be fulfilling. We assume that good sexual chemistry that leads to fulfilling sex will meet our intimacy needs and get rid of emotional loneliness and trauma flashbacks. However, sex cannot rescue us. Sex is a practice and sexual chemistry is only one of the ingredients. You can't start cooking with the assumption that the ingredients themselves will create flavour. It is the act of cooking that creates the right flavour, texture and taste.

However, because we are not taught to see sex as an active practice that one needs to invest time to learn about—especially if one has experienced trauma of some sort—we fall prey to many unrealistic expectations. Casual sex (engaging in physical sexual acts without any expectations of commitment) brings a certain style of attachment and a specific way of relating to the world. The practice of polyamory (dating more than one person at once, openly) brings with it its own patterns of attachment that people who practise monogamy find difficult to understand. Asexuality or celibacy are orientations that create attachment styles of their own. There is no one right way to create a meaningful life of secure attachment for yourself.

When we view sexuality (including the choice to not be sexual) as a natural, fluid and essential part of our life, our relationship with the world expands. When the sex is suffering in your relationship, inquire about the connection itself. Have there been breaks in trust? Do you feel a loss of respect? Are there inconsistencies or hidden needs between you and your partner(s) that have not been voiced out? That's where the key to sexual intimacy is: it is in strengthening your connection to your partner.

## Conflict transformation is the key to relationship maturity

Loving partners also shut down sexually with each other from time to time. They feel new kinks and desires in their own masturbation rituals and their libidos mismatch, conflicts happen and new ways of being together emerge. This is also normal. In fact, it is only through welcoming change that love deepens over time and moves from its infantile stages of infatuation into a more mature and solid partnership. This cannot happen without learning how to fight well, fight fairly and transform conflict into medicine.

People take months to understand their own triggers and change old habits. We fail six times at things even when we know how to do them well, before we suddenly succeed the seventh time—and even this is normal. Bindu and Rajeev are a great example of a couple building an inner work *practice* together. They created tenderness for each other's trauma history, attachment styles and mistakes, even though they started at a place of judgement, blame and shutting down.

Often one can get very challenged by watching others perform their acts of love and unity on social media. Curated screens propagate the fantasy that love is only true when it is displayed in its infantile stage, full of beautiful vacations, hot sex and dramatic proposals. This makes people think of themselves as failing partners when the relationship naturally begins to deepen with time and familiarity and moves away from the early stages.

This harmful, shaming narrative that 'the right kind of love will feel easy' misses the consistency of everyday work—the real labour required to be put in by partners to create and maintain a safe, flowing, deep space of open-hearted connection together, year after year.

*Bindu and Rajeev feel like the elements of water and earth. With the right perspective towards each other's complementary strengths and weaknesses, they have the capacity to create a solid, loving nest of support for one another.'*

Notes to myself in my art therapy journal after a session with Bindu and Rajeev.

## Chapter Takeaways

Long-term relationships bring out our trauma histories, which often include our triggers and conflict styles. When conflict escalates, intimacy weakens and makes way for shame, anger, fear of abandonment and other painful feelings.

## Exercise 7: **Understand your shame spiral in relationships**

As you read, in this chapter, we sank our teeth into the issue of sexual disconnection in marriage. For many older generations, this concept is normalized as 'that is just how it is' in public Indian discourse. We learnt about the lives of Bindu and Rajeev, a cis-straight couple who took bold steps towards more connection with each other in sex therapy. By negotiating life's complex challenges together, they gave their families a lot of support and care—but in the process, they lost access to each other's hearts, bodies and spirits. However, despite years of discord, they could heal the built-up shame in their relationship.

Perhaps this chapter may have prompted you to think about where you're experiencing disconnection in your own relationships, and how running away from conflict and not participating in quick and adequate repair may have led to your relationships suffering. If it did, consider the following for your journal.

Make sure you're in a relaxed state of mind. You can lie next to your partner, or by yourself, and write or reflect:

- Do you know how you feel when you experience shame in your body? (Refer to exercises in Chapter 1.)

........................................................................................

........................................................................................

........................................................................................

........................................................................................

........................................................................................

........................................................................................

........................................................................................

........................................................................................

........................................................................................

........................................................................................

........................................................................................

........................................................................................

........................................................................................

........................................................................................

- When you experience a conflict with your partner, where does your mind take you?

........................................................................................

........................................................................................

........................................................................................

........................................................................................

........................................................................................

...........................................................................................................

...........................................................................................................

...........................................................................................................

...........................................................................................................

...........................................................................................................

...........................................................................................................

...........................................................................................................

...........................................................................................................

...........................................................................................................

...........................................................................................................

...........................................................................................................

...........................................................................................................

- Write 'I feel most ashamed when my partner says _____ about me'

...........................................................................................................

...........................................................................................................

...........................................................................................................

...........................................................................................................

...........................................................................................................

...........................................................................................................

...........................................................................................................

...........................................................................................................

...............................................................................................

...............................................................................................

...............................................................................................

...............................................................................................

...............................................................................................

...............................................................................................

...............................................................................................

...............................................................................................

...............................................................................................

- Journal about this for ten minutes.

...............................................................................................

...............................................................................................

...............................................................................................

...............................................................................................

...............................................................................................

...............................................................................................

...............................................................................................

...............................................................................................

...............................................................................................

........................................................................

........................................................................

........................................................................

........................................................................

........................................................................

........................................................................

........................................................................

........................................................................

........................................................................

........................................................................

........................................................................

........................................................................

........................................................................

........................................................................

........................................................................

........................................................................

........................................................................

........................................................................

Notice if you experience flashbacks of any fights your parents may
have had. Try to focus on any or all of the following questions.
Take it slow and give your body time and space to experience each
question fully.

- What were you doing at the times when your parents were having a bad fight?

..............................................................................................................

..............................................................................................................

..............................................................................................................

..............................................................................................................

..............................................................................................................

..............................................................................................................

- Where were your siblings?

..............................................................................................................

..............................................................................................................

..............................................................................................................

..............................................................................................................

..............................................................................................................

- Where were your friends?

..............................................................................................................

..............................................................................................................

..............................................................................................................

..............................................................................................................

..............................................................................................................

..............................................................................................................

- Who took care of you during their fight?

.............................................................................................

.............................................................................................

.............................................................................................

.............................................................................................

.............................................................................................

- Who took care of you after their fight?

.............................................................................................

.............................................................................................

.............................................................................................

.............................................................................................

.............................................................................................

- Did you see them reconcile? What was that experience like?

.............................................................................................

.............................................................................................

.............................................................................................

.............................................................................................

.............................................................................................

- If not, write down some of the things your parents or early caregivers did after a fight. For example: 'My parents gave each other the silent treatment for a few days after a nasty fight'; or 'My parents disappeared into their room and acted like nothing happened the next day, and us children remained confused'.

........................................................................................

........................................................................................

........................................................................................

........................................................................................

........................................................................................

........................................................................................

........................................................................................

## Something to consider as you're writing

These behaviours that your parents displayed with the limited knowledge they probably had at the time could have had an impact on your own psychological beliefs about the role of conflict in relationships. Many of us were taught to fight dirty and never repair, and so we never got an opportunity to explore the depth of our beliefs about what we think long-term love should look, sound and feel like. Others may have seen their parents fight without a clear end, and so they may have internalized the idea that boundaries are selfish and mean that our partner doesn't love us enough to keep continuing the fight with the same intensity.

Sometimes, we might think that 'working' on a relationship is bad or dreary and that if something is naturally good, then it shouldn't include work. We may believe that if a romance is meant to be, it should feel easy and non-triggering. Nothing could be further from the truth. If you want to create a relationship of intention, then putting in the work is an early and a consistent form of investment.

- Do you harbour a fantasy that a long-term relationship should be mostly easy, flowing and positive and not push your shame buttons?
- Think back to where you learnt this.
- Now, consider what this belief or any connected beliefs do to how you behave in your own relationships.

## Exercise 8: Map your trauma responses in relationship conflict

Trauma responses are responses our body comes up with to protect us from threat. These are not entirely in our control, but becoming aware of our trauma responses and giving our body the safety it needs when it feels threatened can help relax us during conflict with a loved one. It can help us turn towards the perceived threat that we experience in a fight with more compassion than constriction.

**Consider the following trauma responses and the ways they are displayed especially during relationship conflict:**

**Fight:** The fight trauma response involves a release of hormones (primarily cortisol and adrenaline) in the body that trigger a reaction to stay and ward off or 'fight' the apparent threat. When we experience the fight response, we display it in these ways during the threat of conflict:

- Crying
- An urge to physically attack through punching, kicking or other methods
- A tight jaw or grinding teeth
- The urge to act immediately

- Glaring at others
- Yelling or speaking with anger
- A feeling of intense anger
- Upset stomach
- Rapid breathing or heart rate
- Tense muscles

**Flight:** The flight trauma response involves a release of stress hormones that signal us to flee from the danger or threat. Instead of staying in a dangerous situation, this response prompts us to run—literally or metaphorically. When we experience the flight response, we display it in these ways during the threat of conflict:

- Restless legs
- Dilated eyes
- Feelings of hypervigilance
- Running away or feeling the urge to run away
- Fidgeting
- Tense jaw
- A feeling of being trapped
- Fear or anxiety
- A feeling of shock, surprise or confusion
- Avoidance

**Freeze:** The freeze trauma response leaves us temporarily paralyzed by fear and unable to move. In this response, rather than fighting off the danger or running away from it, we do nothing; the perceived threat causes a hypotonic or immobile reaction. Someone in a freeze response may experience numbness or a sense of dread. When we experience the freeze response, we display it in these ways during the threat of conflict:

- Feeling cold
- Numbness in the body
- Pale skin
- Feeling heavy or stiff
- A sense of fear, anxiety or dread
- A pounding heart
- Decreased heart rate
- Dissociation (feeling as if you're outside of your body)

**Fawn:** The fawn response involves complying after the fight, flight or freeze responses failed. This response to a threat is common for people who have experienced abuse, especially those with narcissistic caregivers or romantic partners.

The fawn response may show up as people-pleasing, even to your detriment. You may use compliance and helpfulness to avoid abuse; you disregard your happiness and well-being no matter how poorly someone treats you. This trauma response is often used to diffuse conflict and return to a feeling of safety. When we fawn, we tend to:

- People-please even when it hurts us
- Comply with whatever the other person wants just to end the conversation or to avoid abuse

*Now that you know the different trauma responses, bring yourself in the picture and answer the following questions:*

- What is your go-to trauma response when you're triggered in conflict with someone close to you?

- How do you feel when you're embodying this trauma response? List some signs in your body that you can remember.

- Now that you're more aware of your responses and your body's signals, think of what brings you out of fight/flight/ freeze or fawn. When I'm in my 'fight response', I like to go to my art studio and play with clay. It helps relax my body and provides an appropriate outlet for the anger that wants to get discharged.

- What helps you?

*Now, write your answers for each trauma response in this table below:*

| Trauma Response | How I feel when I am in this trauma response | Steps I can take to gently bring myself out of this response | Things I want to remind myself of the next time I'm in this trauma response |
|---|---|---|---|
| Fight | Example:<br><br>When I'm in fight mode, I feel:<br>Angry, mean, rude and vengeful | • Go for a walk<br>• Paint<br>• Work with pottery and pound clay in my art room | • I am allowed to feel angry<br>• My feelings are okay.<br>• I am not allowed to hurt my partner when I'm angry.<br>• I will wait for 20 mins and express my feelings once I'm feeling less angry. |

| Flight | | | |
|--------|--|--|--|
| Freeze | | | |
| Fawn | | | |

Congratulations, you've made yourself aware of what is generally extremely difficult to list out. Give yourself a pat on the back! Consider sharing your answers with your partner/loved one next, or even doing this exercise with them. This exercise can serve as a helpful relationship reflection activity and create shared vulnerability in your connection.

## Exercise 9: Create co-regulation spaces with your loved ones

Healthy skills that are related to intimacy cannot be learnt in selfish or one-sided relationship dynamics. They must be learnt and practised in mutually reciprocal relationships where each partner is doing their part to create security and growth.

A trauma-informed partnership is one where partners actively choose their relationship to be a 'container' of their growth. This means that in a partnership like this, both partners welcome the natural challenges of being with someone and use those challenges and opportunities to deepen their understanding of each other's patterns, needs, histories and hopes.

As partners do this, instead of turning away, they turn towards each other. This is called co-regulation.

Co-regulation is not co-dependency. In the latter type of relationship, partners depend on the other person to change and get stuck in rigid roles of relating. The rescuer waits for the damsel-in-distress to become less distressed so that he can express what he needs, or the angry teacher corrects and overcorrects the backbencher partner only to end up completely disconnected from her own needs. Co-regulation is about interdependence and safety. It's creating a space where both partners can say without doubt, 'I trust you enough to know that we have each other's back. I trust you to correct me when I'm wrong or to help me when I'm struggling and I know you feel similarly about me.'

As people living and loving in urban India, we are experiencing our relationship culture and the expectations and needs of our partners and our families shift at speeds like never before. Perhaps this chapter may have prompted you to think about where you're experiencing disconnection in your own relationships.

## If it did, consider the following questions:

- What are some ways in which you and your partner, friend, family member or companion regulate yourselves when life feels fast or hard?
- Do you soothe each other, or are you more inclined to doing this alone in your own time and space?
- How does this impact your partner?
- Does your partnership have a solid, metaphorical 'home' that you both come back to when life feels hard? If not, could you both create it together?

## Somatic ways to create these safe spaces together

Co-regulation is not just an intellectual process of talking about connection. It is about feeling connected together. For this to become more of a reality in your relationship, please consider these somatic, body-based rituals of connection in partnership:

- Disconnect from your phones half an hour before going to bed. Keep the phones in another room. Take an oil or lotion you both like and slowly massage each other. While you're doing so, ask your partner questions about their inner world.
- Sit across from each other and hold each other's hands. This might feel uncomfortable or silly at first. Count to five and sync your breathing with your partner. Open your eyes and embrace. If words come, allow them to surface.
- Slowly lie down next to each other and experience the sensation of feeling more in-tune, more in-sync. Our breath is the key to our hearts. As you're breathing softly and with more awareness, hold each other in bed and create time to cuddle with no agenda for the next fifteen minutes.

## Some suggested questions:

- What feels good to you about life these days?
- What have you been worried about?
- What have you been thinking about this week?
- How are you feeling about your body today? Where does it hurt? Where does it feel good?
- What would you like to share with me? I'm feeling open to hearing about what's happening in your heart these days.

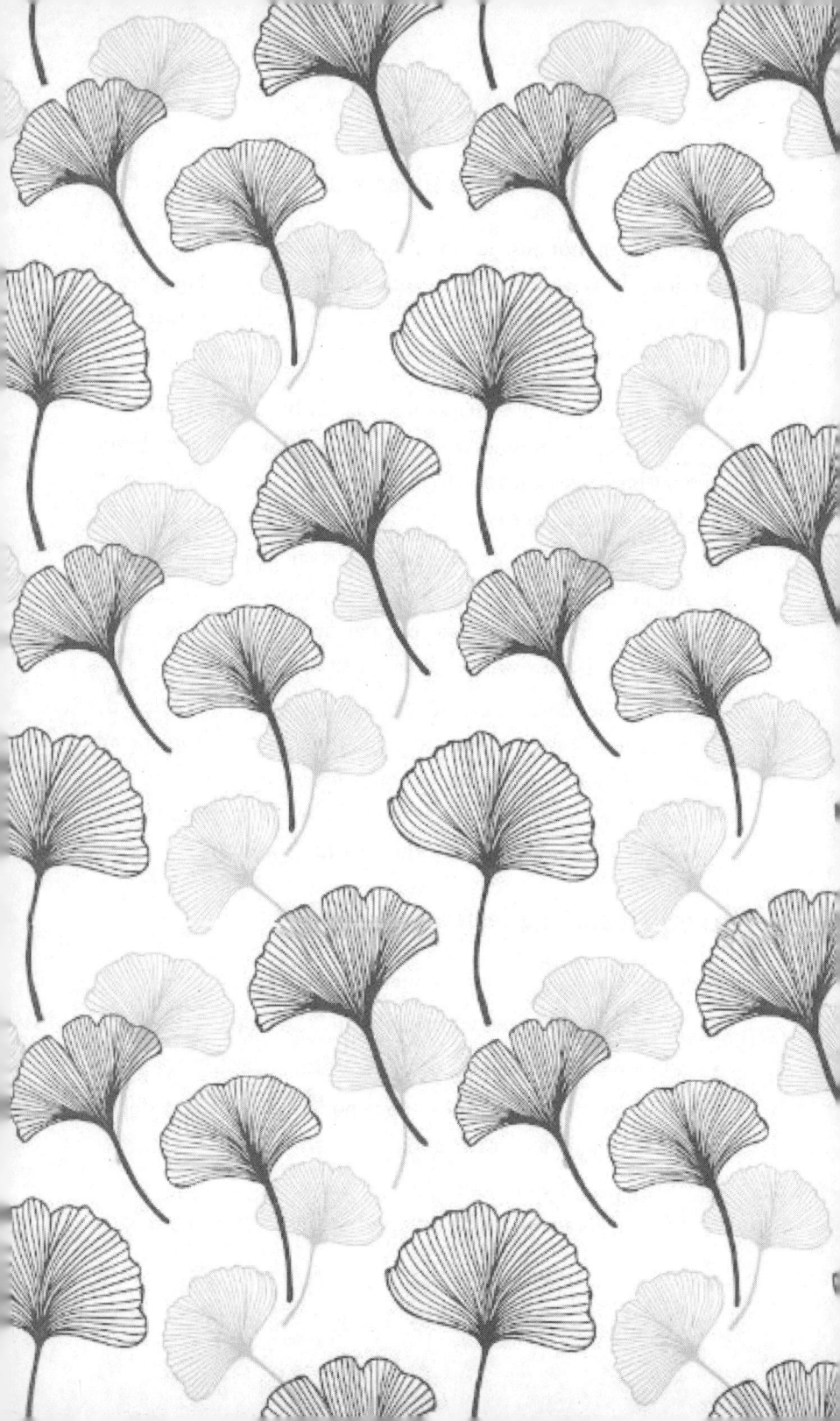

# PART 3

# Deepen

*Where does shame come from?*

*'Everything you judge about yourself served a purpose at the time'*

—*Dr Gabor Maté, trauma-informed physician*

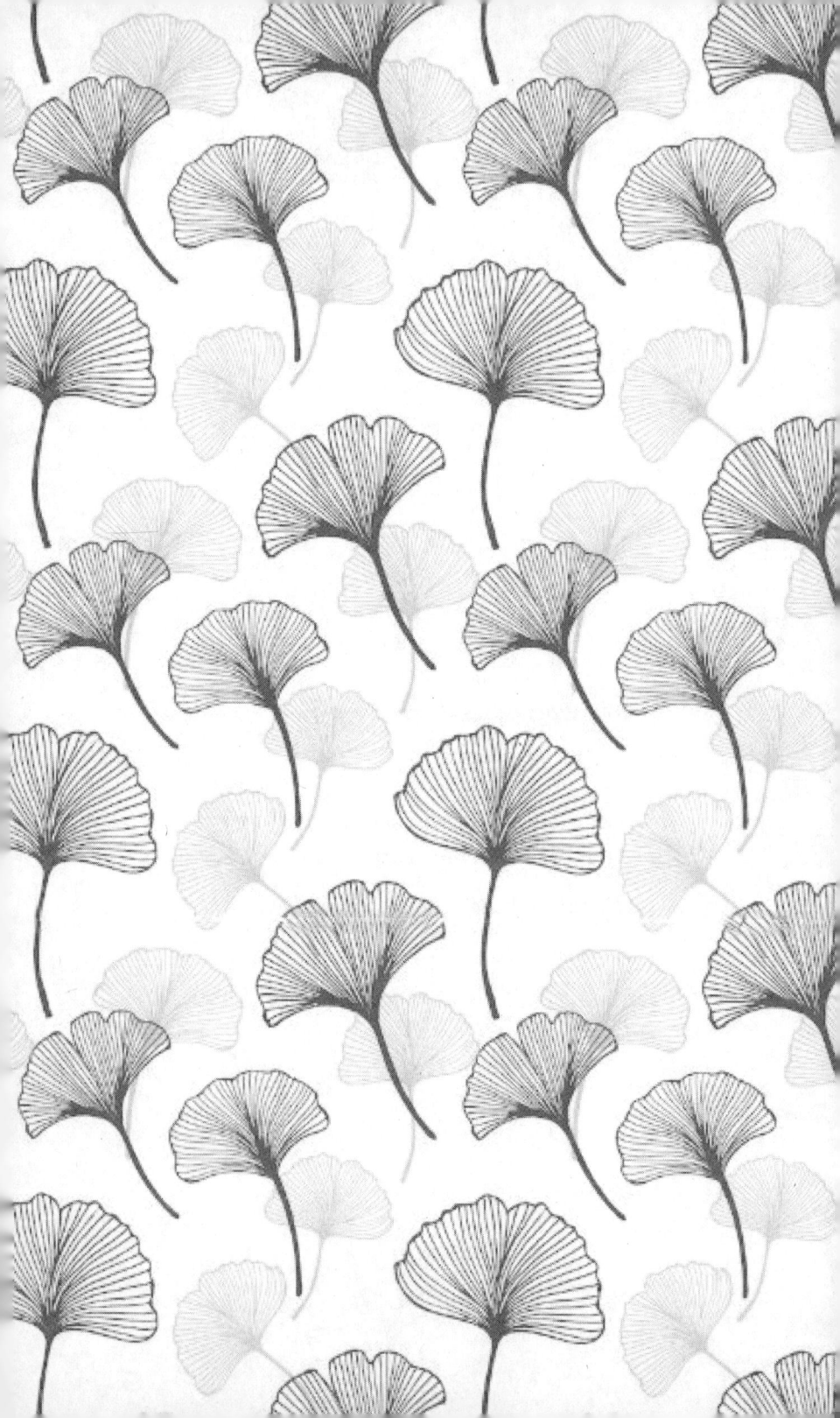

# CHAPTER 5

# 'Shame, shame, puppy shame, all the monkeys know your name!'

## On schools, bullying, isolation and the roots of sexual shame

Rahul had been tender-hearted as an adolescent. He would offer to share his tiffin with his classmates when his mother packed cheese sandwiches instead of the usual rajma-chawal. He would cry easily when a meaner kid called him a name and he would say yes to his teacher's orders even if he didn't know what they meant. 'What would you say is your earliest memory of feeling deeply ashamed of your body, Rahul?' I asked the gentle, nervous man who sat by me. Rahul was now thirty-three.

'In biology class ... I think,' he replied before going on to narrate what felt like an experience no young adult should ever go through. This is an experience that perhaps many of us may have even encountered in our own schools when we were in the sixth or seventh grade, one that may not even have registered as anything other than slightly funny. However, like in so many such events, the person who was impacted by it may remember it quite differently.

One hot summer's day at a busy school in New Delhi, Ms Sheela, the school's Biology teacher, was teaching class 6-A the reproductive system—with all its complex scientific names that Rahul said none of his friends understood. He recalled that most kids in that classroom were too busy giggling at how uncomfortable Ms Sheela looked, and some kids would try and ask the most inappropriate questions to rile her up for adolescent kicks. Sneering glances were being exchanged by the students; notes and chits with lewd jokes were being abundantly passed around.

When the teacher was explaining the menstrual cycle with a funny little diagram, eleven-year-old Rahul experienced what he now knows was his first-ever erection in class. Completely embarrassed, he confessed he had no idea why he was feeling this rush of blood in his penis—he wasn't turned on by anything or anyone that he could think of. Yet, his pants were obviously bulging at the crotch. Rahul was clueless about what to do and tried to cover it up till the end of that period. He thought he would go to the bathroom when the class ended to understand what his body was doing.

Unfortunately for him, the teacher happened to see Rahul fidget in his seat and glance towards the door. Misunderstanding his distracted, restless body language for inattention and disobedience, and perhaps already angered by the sneers she was getting at her discomfort with the topic, she asked Rahul to stand up and answer a question that she had just posed to the class.

Not knowing how to say no, Rahul stood, but asked for permission to go to the toilet. An ill-trained Ms Sheela was shocked to see his bulging crotch and took this young student's blossoming sexuality as a personal offense. She shamed Rahul in front of the whole class for being a 'lewd, dirty boy with no manners'. 'How dare you even do this in class?' she scolded. 'You do not respect me, you sick boy!'

The school should have created a safe environment where young people were given the right circumstances in which to understand their sexuality and taught the children the appropriate terminology and social protocol around masturbation. They could have hired professional sex educators or even doctors with training to hold sex-ed workshops. Instead, this school, like so many in our country, evidently believed in instilling shame as punishment for what they perceived as disobedient, vulgar behaviour.

The entire class fell silent as a very triggered Ms Sheela kept screaming at Rahul, accusing him of having 'dirty thoughts'. She eventually asked him to leave the class. Instead of offering healthy, mature education on human sexuality, Ms Sheela had punished an eleven-year-old boy's natural, healthy, age-appropriate physical experience.

Sitting in my office all these years later, Rahul recalled his shame-inducing punishment with tears in his eyes. His body was closed, the atmosphere heavy; it was clear he hadn't talked about this in years. 'I had to write "I am a dirty boy and I will respect my brothers and sisters" one hundred times on the class board in Hindi and English, and I did not even know what I had done wrong,' he recalled. 'I just remember hating my penis, slapping that part of my body, crying for long hours and worrying that my friends and parents will now think that I'm a sick monster.' Sadly, the experience did not end there.

Rahul received no reassurances and no one told him that he had done nothing wrong. Upon reaching home, Rahul discovered that his parents had been called to the principal's office to discuss Rahul's 'lewd behaviour'. He remembers being severely beaten with his dad's belt that entire month. 'How dare you stare at a teacher?' his father would demand to know. 'Is this what we have taught you? Is this what you do when we think you are studying?' Each time Rahul would start bawling or try to defend himself, the word *'nalayak'* (useless boy!) would be yelled at him, along with '*Ladki jaise kaun rota hain teri umar mein?*' (Which boy cries like a girl at your age?)

Years later, at the age of thirty-three, Rahul experienced a problem he found very confusing. He enjoyed sexual intimacy with his partner, whom he loved and felt attracted towards—that is, until they began to fight. On weeks when the conflicts between them escalated and spiralled and mean words were said, Rahul said he experienced a total lack of libido. He was horrified at having erectile dysfunction in his thirties and losing all connection to his penis.

'What do you do when this happens?' I asked him.

'I feel really, really scared, and rush to watch at least an hour of porn to get some feeling back there,' he replied. 'I sometimes slap that part of my body ... like I used to when I was eleven, I guess ... and I just hate myself for it.'

He wondered if he was aging or if he had overstimulated himself with graphic imagery. He was also concerned about having lost interest in his partner and that what he believed about himself deep down was true—that his penis might be 'broken'.

Rahul and I worked together for two years. When he first accessed therapy, it was for his general anxiety in relationships—he wanted to learn ways in which he could feel more present in his relationship and not catastrophize that it would end each time he fought with his partner. In the first year of his treatment, Rahul proved himself to be a stellar psychotherapy client. He came to therapy on time each week and was consistent with out-of-session reflection and writing. He often complimented me on my ways of motivating him: 'You're a great teacher,' he would say. He would use his mind to sit with the complex psychotherapy concepts that I would explain to him and would report positive results very quickly.

I was somewhat sceptical of his need to be an all-star client with no conflicts whatsoever. However, I waited for the process to unfold the deeper layers of his reality in their own time. It was only after the first year of solid work, when he thought he was 'healed', that Rahul hesitantly brought up his penis shame as one last thing to work on. I found this moment to be a pivotal one in our alliance. I told him that I was so thrilled that he had felt safe enough to trust me with this very vulnerable part of himself, and that I was looking forward to supporting him in understanding this aspect of his life.

At first, Rahul did not like what I said. 'What do you mean, Neha?' he asked. 'Haven't I already been so vulnerable? Don't you feel I trust you enough?' This was one of the first times Rahul had allowed his deeply hidden defences to surface—he was angry with me. After that, I began opening our therapy sessions with soothing sentences of affirmation for his sexuality. 'Your anger is welcome here,' I told him. 'You don't have to be perfect here. Tell me more about this anger, Rahul—who are you angry with?' Rahul's body unleashed a flood of overpowering emotion in a way that I had not seen before.

'So, wanting to talk about my penis, and how I hate that I can't connect to it—doesn't that make me a monster?' he would ask at least once every month.

'It makes you a brave, tender-hearted and honest human, Rahul, who cares so much about his partner,' I would reply. 'I am so proud of your courage to understand yourself.'

He would then cry for ten minutes. This emotional connection opened something powerful in Rahul's nervous system.

He had needed to trust someone in authority—someone who, unlike Ms Sheela, would not shame his display of his vulnerabilities. Over time, this would give him permission to reframe the shame-filled beliefs he still nurtured because of his teacher's bullying. He had not understood it but an authority figure had let him down and impacted his sense of self at an age when he should have had reassuring parental and educator-led guidance.

Rahul spent months working through caring for his shame and rebuilding his connection to a vulnerable body part. Years later, he told me that hearing his therapist say 'Your tears are so honest and they are always welcome here' at the end of every session was a powerful reminder for him to try and internalize that anti-shame affirmation for himself.

He was not weak for feeling so powerfully, nor was he weak for being tender-hearted and believing the degrading words of his unkind teacher. He had just been a gentle child who had had the misfortune of experiencing a traumatic, abusive public humiliation. Now, as an adult, he has the power to be his own inner authority with gentle guidance from those he trusts.

## Sexual shame can lead to emotional disconnection

If we analyse in-depth, there are subtle yet powerful links between our sexual desires— that which makes us feel good—and this emotion called shame that makes us feel bad. We might be able to see the complication of this mixture for ourselves.

Shame is technically a parasympathetic pause in our nervous system. Translated into language that isn't neurobiology focused, it is most commonly described in the therapy world as a negative self-conscious emotion. This means that it is a negative type of emotion that makes a person feel conscious of themselves in such a way that it blocks that person from feeling good about themselves.

When researchers study shame in trauma studies, they track two areas of the brain: the *prefrontal cortex*, an area dedicated to moral reasoning; and the *posterior insula*, an area that triggers the visceral response of disgust. When most people feel shame—which by definition is an intense and strong feeling—it strikes our body's understanding of morals and evokes a feeling of disgust or repulsion in ourselves.

Can you see why so many of us naturally want to hit the escape button the moment we feel this emotion even in small ways? Can you see how our bodies might shut themselves down when this emotion shows up, as in Rahul's case above or in Kusha's in Chapter 1? Furthermore, when we overlap the most vulnerable parts of our human system—our intimate sexual parts, kinks, fantasies, desires and needs—with the most negative messaging, we create this potent mix of terrible self-hatred towards something that is supposed to make us feel good about ourselves.

## Chapter Takeaways

Remember that sexual shame is both an old and often a hidden emotion, which stems from having been shamed, directly or indirectly. We pick up shaming messages from different parts of our childhood including our families and our school systems. If we had severely traumatizing experiences in school, chances are we still carry some shame from those into our adult lives. There is no one specific formula to reframe all types of sexual shame, but it helps to know this key fact about ourselves and our loved ones: what each human body perceives as harmful depends a lot on that particular body's trauma history.

## Exercise 10: Create your own trauma timeline

A trauma timeline is a map where we can see the links between experiences. We often make timelines of our professional milestones—graduating college, getting a job, receiving an award, etcetera. Similarly, there's something called a trauma timeline—to map incidents, big or small, that have been sources of trauma for us.

What you feel sensitive about or hurt by depends on your own trauma history, and each person is allowed that freedom in a mature, healthy society. Our social identities are part of that trauma history.

For example, if you were designated female at birth and grew up accepting that identity (this is called being cisgender) and have lived your life as a woman, you would have probably experienced a specific set of systemic traumas. Your trauma timeline could include common female experiences of being shamed at school that were normalized in our colonial education systems—such as having the length of your skirt publicly measured during morning assembly as a test of 'appropriateness' by the class prefect or being told you by a teacher or a parent that you are 'asking to be slut shamed' because your bra-strap was showing. Maybe you were continuously policed by an overprotective mother to 'sit like a day' with your legs crossed, even beyond the realm of social etiquette, while a male member of your family wasn't expected to be half as self-conscious at all times at home. Perhaps, like many women, this makes you unable to fully relax even in the safe company of your intimate partner.

Your timeline could also include more severely harmful experiences of shame: incidents of sexual violence, interpersonal harm, being publicly shamed for your body or your choice of dress, having your whereabouts policed, not receiving guidance about menstrual health or being put down for having sexually liberal views.

### How to create a trauma timeline

Choose a day when you have at least two hours for this exercise. It could be a holiday that you're spending by yourself, not surrounded by family and friends.

- Start with your earliest memory of shame in your body. When was the earliest time someone shamed you and for what? Go as far back as you can remember, without forcing yourself to excavate something that might be buried for its own reasons.

- If there's a big incident in your life that made you feel grief, shock, terror or helplessness and shook your sense of self in a large way—examples include domestic violence, early death or divorce of parents, rape, shooting or natural disaster—consider mapping that as 'big T' trauma.

- Now, consider events or an ongoing event in your life that caused some amount of fear, distress or helplessness. This may be something like an abrupt breakup or some other relationship challenge, loss of a job or financial worries. While these likely didn't threaten your sense of self, they perhaps caused anxiety, depression or other significant negative effects. Consider mapping these as 'small t' trauma.

- Small t trauma can create the same symptoms as big T trauma does—although they are usually less severe. If you've already been in therapy or inner work process, this should be easy to name. If not, this might be a bit harder to remember. Know that we cannot understand something that we avoid, and all parts of us deserve our own understanding. We cannot expect someone else to know these parts of us if we have not confronted them and tried to understand them ourselves.

- Create a dot and label this memory.

- Now, create a timeline of your traumas around shame.

- Label each memory with dates, years, names of people who were involved in that incident if you feel like.

- Once you're done with creating a timeline of this information, take a pause and practise belly breathing as we've done in the previous chapters.

- When you feel ready, revisit this timeline, and try to answer these questions for each memory: What did I feel in my body at that time? What did I do about that feeling? Where is this feeling now in my body?

As you engage with this difficult but important reflection, you may feel activated, triggered or taken back in time. Allow these feelings to arise, and make ample space to write about them. If you have a person you can trust, try telling them about your feelings if you feel like it. Remember, the more we practise talking to others about what we find hard, the easier it becomes to talk to ourselves with gentleness and compassion. Our inner voice strengthens with practise.

# CHAPTER 6

# 'Shhh ... don't do so much drama, okay?'

*On sexual violence, abusive relationships and the shame of trauma bonds*

When I was a teenager growing up in Hyderabad, pornography was just starting to become freely available to anyone with an internet connection. At the time, owning a personal computer was a luxury for middle-class Indians. The weird, shrill dial-up sounds of the internet connecting was a regular phenomenon in the 1990s. However, Fiza—a twenty-two-year-old queer artist living in Bombay—was part of a newer generation that had had access to the internet even before hitting puberty. Thus, she had attained exposure to queer subcultures, digital erotic culture, cosplay culture and the free-thinking corners of the internet from a very young age.

When Fiza approached me for a session, she seemed very open, accepting and aware of what therapy was. She even had some curiosity about what sexuality-focused art therapy might entail. Fiza told me that she came from a family environment that had ensured she was aware of the dangers of too much time spent online, especially with the darker subcultures of the internet that are not child-friendly.

She spoke of her mother's forward-thinking, harm-reduction approach as a parent very fondly, and even recalled conversations between her parents in which her mother scolded her father for not reading up on a new trending topic or something in the news. Fiza was fortunate to have early childhood and adolescent experiences that were made emotionally safe by parents who educated themselves about a changing world and created a nurturing home atmosphere.

Therapy becomes a joyful, deep, alive and pleasurable experience when working with such individuals. With secure attachment in the relationship, the client looks forward to building trust with a 'good-enough' therapist who is a 'good-enough' match, and any therapeutic conflicts and triggers that organically arise are safely worked through within the boundaries of this trusted relationship. In myriad ways, our childhood can impact the trajectories of our entire lives. In cases where many of us where we may not have had the good fortune of a safe early childhood, like Fiza had, we might have to work that much harder to change our core fears, understand our triggers and then take the brave steps towards creating a life of joy, trust and abundance.

But all was not going well for Fiza when she came to see me. She was struggling with a bizarre, unsettling experience with her boyfriend of two years, Raghav, who was very accepting of her queerness. She found this to be a very endearing quality of Raghav, to accept her for who she was. It is surprising to me when it comes as a shock to many heterosexual Indian people that bisexual people can be in fulfilling relationships with people of the opposite gender identity, and still identify as bisexual. Bisexuality does not get erased when one is in a seemingly heterosexual relationship. Women who identify as bisexual often tell me that being partnered with an emotionally-intelligent male partner who knows about their sexual orientation helps them live a less shame-filled existence, and that such partners are rare to find. Indian society has some work to do to be able to decolonize itself from the concept of sexual binaryness and to embrace the concept of sexual fluidity.

Fiza, however, had a different problem at hand. She revealed that he had recently confessed that he was unable to feel attracted to her and had been using over-the-counter medication to sustain an erection. Raghav was twenty-three and was working a job that kept him on his feet for several hours a day. When he returned home, he was so fatigued that all he wanted to do was drink and watch TV. The fatigue had worsened over the last three months.

Fiza told me that she liked his dry sense of humour, but lately his jokes had become cruder and more sarcastic and even their friends were getting concerned about Raghav's callous behaviour. The previous weekend, Raghav got extremely drunk at a friend's birthday party. Instead of going to sleep in the room Fiza was sleeping in, he found himself passed out next to Fiza's best friend, Sahiti. The friend later stormed out of the house in the middle of the night saying that she had been molested by Raghav.

Later, in a group text to their friends, Sahiti declared that she had been groped by a very drunk Raghav and as a result she had decided to cut him off from her life. She also texted Fiza advising her to get out of this relationship quickly because Raghav was a potential rapist, and, in Sahiti's eyes, the relationship was a disaster in the making. When confronted about these allegations, Raghav told Fiza that he remembers groping someone's thighs aggressively in his drunken stupor before falling asleep. However, he claimed he thought it was Fiza.

Raghav took offense to Sahiti's text and replied to the group saying, 'Sorry I was so drunk that I didn't know who I was touching, but don't do so much drama, okay? Everyone was drunk anyway, stop being a tightass.' This is when Fiza decided to seek professional help. She was terribly upset at her boyfriend's creepy behaviour, but more than that she was triggered by his complete dismissal of the intensity of what he had done. Fiza also saw herself as a committed, loyal, caring girlfriend who was interested in supporting her boyfriend to seek help. She decided to take a short break from their relationship with the hope that Raghav would confront his abusive behaviour and make a change.

I met Fiza twice before she came together with Raghav for a couples' therapy session. The mood in the session was understandably tense, and both Fiza and Raghav seemed distant, anxious and slightly closed-off. Traditional couples' therapy advice is that therapists should resist asking couples for the truth too early in the session, because it could scare people off. However, I trained under two supervisors and mentors who were advocates of truth-telling early, especially when there are patterns of abuse involved in the relationship in question.

When I started deepening my studies in couples' and group therapy, I interned at a therapy centre for rape survivors in Chicago. I witnessed the power of not playing it safe in the therapy room and instead nudging my clients—especially those who have a history of abuse—to gain the confidence to speak their deepest truths early. From couples' therapist Terry Real, I learnt the art of 'joining' with the couple in their truth through practices of radical and upfront honesty.

Of course, this is a challenging task for people who believe that therapy should be a safe space where they can expect to not only be validated but also coddled so that they can feel 'safe-enough' to express themselves. While safety is very important and foundational, safety without focusing on truth-telling as a value can enable people with a history of abusive behaviour to continue to hide, lie and remain untruthful to the therapist, to their partner and to themselves. Because I often go against this notion of safety only, I practise creating 'brave spaces' instead, where courage is encouraged early on and clients experience some defensiveness in themselves at first.

Raghav had perhaps heard from Fiza that I would challenge him to speak truthfully about what had happened on the night he molested Fiza's best friend. So, when I started the session inviting his narrative into the room, he replied, 'I am sorry for hurting Fiza, but she needs to understand that I was just drunk. I am not a molester or a bad person, and Sahiti has a history of being overly dramatic and sensitive to jokes and small events. Please tell Fiza that I won't hurt her again.'

Fiza grimaced as she heard her boyfriend's insensitive take on his own behaviour. But she forced a smile and said, 'I'm so happy you're saying you won't hurt me again. Thank you for being a good boyfriend. I have told Neha a bit about your past struggles with depression and drinking. Shall I tell her more?' Before Raghav could respond, I set some structure to the session.

'No,' I said. 'I'm sorry, but no. We are not proceeding this way. Fiza, I noticed that you made a face when Raghav was sharing his understanding of the night he molested your best friend—'

'But I didn't molest her, Neha,' Raghav interrupted me loudly. 'Sahiti was also drunk, and she made it all up!'

'This is exactly what we won't do here,' I responded. 'In this therapy room, you're being asked to hold a mirror to your own behaviour. We will let each person finish their point and then speak. We will pause and truly listen, and most importantly ...' I looked at Fiza before continuing, 'we will gather up the courage to speak what's on our minds. Otherwise, we're going to get nowhere.'

Raghav fell silent and brooded for a bit. Fiza looked relieved. Her eyes welled up and she said, 'You're making me see how much I hide what I really want to say.'

Setting structure in couples' trauma work helps maintain a sense of equilibrium in what is essentially a chaotic, messy process of immense emotional labour on the part of the psychotherapist. We can trigger people's resistance to authority, and play against their expectation of 'unconditional positive regard.' Holding a mirror to clients not only helps in radical accountability but also often melts shame and makes space for deeper truths. The skill of a clinician lies in making clients feel that they're being cheered on to undo their own dysfunction without making them feel attacked or threatened.

Fiza did a lot of the talking in that session. She described how she had been lifting a major part of the workload of the relationship and felt that not only was her life imbalanced but also that she was being taken advantage of. Intuitively, she sensed Raghav was lying about not molesting Sahiti. Coming from a family where conversation was encouraged from childhood, Fiza kept pleading with Raghav to be honest. 'I will forgive you,' she wept, 'and I'll work on getting Sahiti to understand that it was a horrible mistake—but please, tell me the truth. Please don't lie.'

Raghav did not seem to understand the pain and confusion Fiza was experiencing. He seemed to have trouble with empathy and consequences. He was used to deflecting his part of the work of their relationship to Fiza, and she was habituated to taking it all on as her problems to fix. Due to her people-pleasing responses to shame, Fiza had been making excuses for him and supporting his missteps at the cost of her friendships. Her desire to be a 'good girlfriend' was so attached to this relationship that she could not see her own part in the toxic cycle that it had become.

Defensiveness is a common response of the nervous system to protect itself. However, if one has been sexually abusive to another, it does not matter if one had been under the influence of alcohol or any other substance. The truth remains that those abusive actions caused someone hurt and harm and traumatized them.

To be in adult relationships, one must behave like an adult, and part of being an adult is to be able to repair the mistakes one makes with genuine intention. One must also be able to handle one's defences because trauma is not an excuse for abuse. Sometimes people tend to claim that anything negative that they did was a result of trauma, and thus it wasn't really their responsibility that it happened. There is a thin line between doing trauma work to understand the causes of one's actions and to repair them, versus using trauma as an excuse to avoid accountability of our actions as adults.

While Fiza and Raghav kept coming to therapy for three weeks after their first session, Raghav became increasingly uninterested in the process. He would partially admit to being aware that he harboured malicious sexual intent towards Sahiti, but he would quickly retract his narrative and change it. Although he was slowly becoming a bit more honest, it came at the cost of causing Fiza severe feelings of pain and confusion in the relationship. However, she was taking leaps forward in seeing how trauma-bonded she was. She experienced a deep desire for a pattern shift and asked for individual sessions.

Fiza started doing less emotional work in their relationship and began voicing her fears as clear asks. She asked Raghav for consistency of narrative as a non-negotiable expectation, without which she would not be with him. In what would become our final session together, Fiza stated that she would no longer invest in couples' therapy nor their relationship if Raghav did not clearly admit what happened that night. She accepted that shifting the state of their relationship was no longer a fantasy. Fiza had come to a straightforward albeit painful realization of her core needs of safety and security.

Raghav promised that he would give her the truth the following week. However, he did not show up to therapy on the promised day. Fiza was gutted that week, but instead of abandoning her own inner-work journey, she started using therapy to turn further inwards. She began to grieve the painful end of her two-year trauma-bonded relationship with Raghav. Slowly, her shame-based feelings of self-worth surfaced in the process. 'Was I not worth even a closure after all that I did for him?' she wept.

Three weeks later, Raghav abruptly came back into Fiza's life, asking for another chance. Fiza, who had just begun giving herself closure, got swept away with her feelings and they ended up having sex. She came into therapy the next day feeling disappointed with herself. 'He is so mean and insensitive, yet I keep going back. Why do I love someone who has been so abusive?'

## Trauma bonds often hit our shame buttons

A trauma bond is a connection between an abusive person and the individual they abuse. The person experiencing abuse may develop sympathy for the abusive person, and even define it as 'unconditional love' for them. Regular relationships become trauma bonds when conflicts escalate, abuse is perpetrated, and instead of sincere repair and healing taking place, the abuse returns, followed by remorse again. This off/on relationship pattern causes immense confusion, anxiety, guilt, shame, loss of a sense of self and activates people's core fears about loss and abandonment, so much so that breaking up and staying broken up feels close to impossible.

Fiza had invested so much of her sense of self in Raghav's recovery that when he returned abruptly without any active change in his abusive behaviour, her desire for receiving soothing and validation from him took her right back into bed with him. This is how strong trauma bonds can be. Fiza's relationship experience is a very good example of how sexual and relationship trauma can impact us at any point in our lives. It is a myth that the answers to all trauma healing lie only in our early childhoods. Some of our most difficult relationships—where we experienced abuse, loss of control, loss of safety, chronic imbalance or violence towards ourselves or someone we cared for—can be extremely traumatizing at any age.

Trauma bonds push the reward and punishment associations in our brain. They keep us wanting to change the other person so that we can finally have the relationship we fantasized about when we met them, but the moment we do get some sort of security with our partner, our punishment centres tell us we should be looking elsewhere for someone better. 'I hate you, but please don't leave me' and 'I love you, but don't get too close to me' can be long-term themes of relationships like these.

The sexual chemistry in relationships like these is typically intense and it can feel like 'true love'. Being in them can feel incredibly shameful because everyone in your life may be advising you to leave for someone better. However, leaving the relationship can feel extremely shame-inducing too, because you are made to feel like the work you put in was not enough to correct the problems. It's a perpetual Catch-22 situation because the partners are bonding with each other based on their sense of inner lack instead of their strengths, shared goals or aligned life perspectives.

Trauma bonding is not 'abnormal', pathological or a disease. It is something many of us do when we're used to imbalanced relationships for whatever reason. It makes sense to look at trauma bonding as a cultural socialization for us Indians. In societies like ours, where caste and gender roles play such a large part in the very structure of relationships, trauma bonds thrive because each partner's self-worth can become attached to their assigned role. Men, however progressive, need to remain in positions of control, while women need to remain nurturing and sweet even if by nature their personality is fierce.

Trauma bonding behaviours exist on a spectrum from minimal (some basic co-dependency) to severe (drastic acts of abuse). A lot of mental health content online does an overly generous job of pathologizing patterns and not a good enough job of helping us understand ourselves within that piece of information or pathology. These relationships can also be so intense because both partners' sense of self-worth is attached to the outcome of the relationship. If they get the other to change, it can feel like they 'won' (the reward centre); but if the partner doesn't change, it can feel like they 'lost' and they need to work harder (the punishment centre).

Instead of focusing on developing a sense of inner security and working on themselves through concrete action steps, the partners promise to change—but that promise is not kept. This can keep them stuck in the waiting game with their sense of self tied in with the chaos of the push and pull until one chooses to break this cycle, just like Fiza did after a year of inner work.

Any bond can be improved if all the people in that bond want to change and put action steps in place to improve. However, it is important to remember that most change takes years of consistent action. Counting on instant change in trauma bonds further worsens this push-and-pull tussle. Some trauma-bonded couples and families who do manage to become more secure and detangle themselves from these patterns do so by:

- Accepting individual responsibility for their harmful behaviour patterns
- Committing to working through their problems together
- Practicing new ways of being together

Other trauma-bonded relationships do not change, even after years of inner work. There isn't one specific formula to mental or sexual health. Everyone has different patterns and the opportunity to change them.

Fiza's shame kept her in people-pleasing mode until she held a mirror to her own behaviours and understood that she was being taken advantage of. She became so obsessed with making her boyfriend a better person that she pleaded with him for accountability, dragged him to therapy and thanked him for basic repair work that any partner should do. Eventually, she lost connection to her own self. It took her time to realize that enabling bad behaviour is also a form of self-abandonment, and most forms of self-abandonment are rooted in our core fears related to shame.

Instead of turning towards our feelings of abandonment and reframing our distorted beliefs about our worth and power, shame makes us control other people: *If I just say yes to what he wants, he will finally love me in the way I need to be loved* or *If I can just push him to apologize, he won't hurt me again next time.* We forget that abusive behaviours are choices, while thoughts and feelings are outside of our control.

Differentiating behaviours and feelings is important, as they tend to be confused. Feelings, whether tied to previous trauma or not, are not something we have control over. Feelings and sensations are transient, like thoughts. They are natural human responses to experiences. For example, we can feel very sad when we miss our abusive ex—the feeling of intense sadness is not in our control. But what we do with this feeling is. If we choose to cry, dance, sing or paint in our ex's memory, we perhaps channel our grief in constructive ways. If we instead end up calling our abusive ex to our home and sleeping with them, we've now intentionally put ourselves in harm's way.

We do have control over the behaviours we choose in response to feelings and experiences. Sometimes, choosing unhealthy or abusive behaviours as a response to hurt feelings becomes so much like second nature to us that it feels like an automatic reaction that is outside of our control. However, it is important to remind yourself that it is not.

## Deal with conflict as it arises, but also know your limits to protect yourself from slipping into cycles of abuse

A person can treat you very well and have a wonderful relationship with you while simultaneously being abusive to someone else in your life and not treating them well at all. Even if you think that they are good to you, they could still be mean to someone else. This is the sad and complicated reality of the human experience. It's important we expand our emotional landscape and learn about the nuances of this human experience instead of adhering to rigid, dysfunctional roles that insist on seeing it as fixed and unmoving.

There is a stereotypical notion that cis-men are naturally non-monogamous, more inclined to be aroused in the morning and prone to masturbate more and cis-women are naturally shy in bed, take time to open up and rarely engage in self-pleasure. Cis-men are always better with money, driving, and small talk, while cis-women are always better with cooking, home decoration and deep conversations. Now if you're someone who has close friends across the gender spectrum, you know that these are falsehoods. These broad stereotypes are examples of fixed views of human existence. They view human beings in terms of the roles they play. Love, too, then becomes the ultimate pedestal of these projected fantasies and ideals. So much of our cinema focuses on glamourizing love stories of extreme sacrifice and giving up everything for the one you love. While this fantasy might feel beautiful and romantic, it is fundamentally unrealistic. This fantasy, until very recently, was sold to us very successfully by mainstream Bollywood cinema. It conditions well-intentioned people like Fiza to fall straight into self-abandonment patterns. How many people are encouraged to remain in abusive marriages in our country because they are taught to believe that 'love means sacrifice'?

The positive aspect of our community-oriented culture is that people are each other's safety nets here. There is a lot of exchange and contact between family members in general, and there are many avenues to depend on—unlike in countries where the people's biggest safety net is their government. However, when people-pleasing becomes compulsive and one starts getting hurt in the process, then our culture and our communities must support individuation. And if they reject us, then we must depend on ourselves and prioritize our wellness. Sexual violence, abuse and trauma are not normal states of every relationship. If you're experiencing these in your own relationships, please find a way to deepen your understanding of the negative impact this could have on you.

Inner work helps us to not be guided by our trauma patterns. It shows us how to discern between choices made from unprocessed trauma and choices made from a state of agency, healing and power. Our nervous systems need trust, compassion, love, mutual care, reciprocity, kindness, gentleness, dependability and more such wonderful feelings consistently to thrive in a world that is inconsistent and chaotic.

When we feel these feelings in the presence of our loved ones even through conflicts, small fights or irritations, we experience what is called 'security'—or secure attachment to that person. This can happen with a friend, a lover, a parent or a teacher. However, the need for these feelings become greater in romantic relationships because the level of physical and emotional intimacy is greater.

We can interpret it as a sign that we are experiencing intense feelings of ambivalence when even after dating a particular person for a while we still do the following:

- Being very judgemental of our partner and their issues as they present themselves in our current reality.
- Being unable to make sense of our contradictory feelings about them and yet continuing to show up for them and then breaking up. The on/off cycle takes centre stage in our connection with them.
- Wanting this person to 'become better' so that when they do that, we can then make our mind up about them.

Can you see how deeply confusing this cycle is? Ambivalence that remains unresolved between partners for a long time corrodes trust, which is the very thing that needs to be strong for relationships to succeed over time. Continued ambivalence makes people's nervous systems feel fearful and unsettled. It creates toxic dynamics of ups and downs of safety and security, which lead to blame, relationship ruptures and fights.

Now, this doesn't mean that you can't be unsure of some things about your lover or that you can't wish that your partner changed some aspects of their weaknesses. Instead, it means that the changes you want in your partner are secondary to your love and acceptance of them as they are. You are willing to choose their burdens as yours and they reciprocate that willingness. Love is work. Love is understanding. Love is deepening your knowledge of how you show up in the world so that others can deepen themselves in your presence.

In a relationship, love is not just about soothing and flowing together. We cannot simply choose to show up when we feel good and are able to. Rather, we have to create a space and work together in a way where as partners we can live a life that is more expansive than the life we can live alone. If our lives aren't better together in the long term, then why choose to create that relationship? Creating such a space takes consistent work. As we saw in Chapter 3, Bindu and Rajeev did a lot of work as a couple to create safety within their relationship, and then did not abuse it.

Please do not mistake conflict for patterns of abuse. Conflict, when navigated well, creates healthy change in partners so that things get easier. Abuse creates distrust and harm in partners so that things get traumatic over time. There is a huge difference between the two. If you've ever been in a truly choice-based, expansive relationship of any sort, you might know what I'm talking about. Think of someone in your life with whom you're very trusting, open and relaxed even when conflict arises. For many people, their therapist is the first person they ever feel this way with. For others, they may feel secure with their sibling or a teacher, a parent or an aunt.

This is not the case in fear-based relationships where people feel 'incomplete' and choose another to understand them or meet them in a way that no one else does. The narrative of 'no one else gets me the way you do so you have to stay with me' is essentially a fear-based narrative. It keeps people stuck even when they have grown out of their choice, and then resentment sets in because the choice has not been renewed, re-examined or worked out together.

When you're with someone for years because you and they choose to expand in the relationship while staying safe and not tearing each other down, your relationship becomes very strong. Relationship strength happens through a process of continuous choice. When two autonomous individuals choose to create more wellness together, this choice is re-examined and refreshed during each phase of life. I wish you the inner work to sustain such an expansiveness in all your relationships.

'Over-functioners often tend to attract under-functioners. With depressed shoulders, Fiza carries the people-pleaser's heavy burden of two and thinks she deserves to; because if she didn't, who would?'

Notes to myself in my therapy journal after a session with Fiza.

## Chapter Takeaways

Sexual and relationship trauma can impact us at any point in our lives, and the shame of trauma bonds is a powerful uncomfortable feeling that requires solid inner work. Some of our most difficult relationships—where we experienced abuse, loss of control, loss of safety, chronic imbalance or violence towards ourselves or someone we cared for—can be extremely traumatizing at any age.

## Exercise 11: *Practise listening to your body's boundaries*

When our bodies tell us we want closeness to someone or something—*even a pet, a cherished object or an idea*—we might feel a sweet, warm, generous feeling inside. Some people feel this close to their heart, while others feel it closer to their stomach. You feel welcome and open. The body relaxes and feels comfortable; it's not edgy about what can go wrong. The body is signalling that it wants to move closer to whatever it is sensing as 'good'.

When our bodies tell us we want distance from something, we might feel a constriction come up. Some people feel this close to their throat and start breathing in a tense, shallow manner around this person, place, animal or thing. Others feel a closing up of their genital area. You feel like leaving and creating distance from that person or thing. You may also feel blocked and shut down. The body is signalling that it wants to move away from whatever it is sensing as 'bad'.

When the body has experienced sexual trauma, has been beaten up with no offer of repair or has been violated in some way, we need to remember that it has been cut off from its own true sensations. The abuser attacked the body and took control of its inner sense of direction, its sense of control and power for that traumatic time. Now imagine if this abuser were someone we once loved and cared for, or someone we still live with and are attached to. This can be very confusing to the traumatized body.

This is how the body loses trust in itself and lives in a state of confusion. If you find your body's sensations living in a constant state of inner conflict, pause for a second and orient your attention towards your inner state. Can you try witnessing it with tenderness? When you start to practise this at first, you might find this very difficult.

Even if the abuser leaves—and even if they left decades ago—
their marks remain. The traumatized body that has not been offered
any repair will often remember how it felt to be abused, even if the
abuser may not remember their acts. Being cut off from one's own
internal sense of direction is a difficult state to live in.

And so, sometimes, the traumatized body may mix up what feels
good and bad all in one. At other times, it might try to create walls
of distance because it is not yet ready to feel open. It may also lean
into over-sharing, over-helping, over-giving or getting very close to
strangers very fast, without having a sense of the boundaries and
structures it needs for it to feel safe, warm, welcome and whole
internally.

*Questions to ponder over:*

- When was the last time you truly felt connected to a loved
  one?
- What did that connection feel like in your body?
- Can you map which parts of your body carry these memories?
- Now think about the times when something felt 'off' to you
  in this connection. How did your body react to this feeling?
  What did you do about it?
- Can you tell when you disbelieve your somatic feelings and
  sensations?

When people reflect on these questions in therapy, some notice
that they're more aware of how often they ignore their body's
language. You might have a similar experience as you think back
to how your body speaks to you. There may have been a time
when you felt disconnected to what was happening inside of you.

You might have felt like ignoring the thoughts and feelings inside of you. It's possible that you felt, 'If I stay with my own feelings too much, I could lose connection with my partner.' These are excellent opportunities to learn your body's communication systems and to teach yourself to believe them as valid information for you to register.

# CHAPTER 7

# 'Sex is great, but when was the last time you truly hugged someone?'

*On touch deprivation and emotional loneliness*

Ramya was forty-one and had lived a unique life. As a highly accomplished academic, she had spent her twenties in and out of research-writing jobs and her thirties completing her PhD and postdoctoral degrees and then teaching in different European countries and India. At forty, she decided to prioritize her love life after being swept off her feet by a charming man her age. He was also an Indian teaching academic but based in the US. She travelled to the United States to visit him and within a few weeks found herself in a heated romance with promises of marriage and children.

Ramya loved babies. Her heart would soar each time her maasi's children visited her parents' flat in Gurgaon. Thus, she abandoned all caution, applied to a teaching position at the same university he taught at and moved to live with him. In another few weeks, the relationship crumbled abruptly as she realized that her partner was already engaged to someone else and had essentially been deceiving both women. As someone who prided herself on her integrity, she cut her ex-partner off and chose to remain as faculty in her new job. She lived by herself in a cozy studio apartment in the middle of town.

When Ramya walked into my therapy office, she carried the aura of a woman who was in tune with her body. This was a woman who seemed like she had access to her inner power and was aware of the impact that her physical appearance and intelligence had on other people. However, as soon she started speaking, I could tell there was a tender, naïve young child inside her, longing to be understood.

'Neha, look—I know sex is great,' she began. 'I've had lots of it and that's not a problem for me. I know you'll say we should all love ourselves and life should be warm and fuzzy and all that jazz. I don't need any sex-positivity lectures from you, please. That's not why I'm here. I'm great at trusting myself and being with myself—I'm not at all like those insecure types who run behind men. I just have a simple question for you: when was the last time you truly hugged someone?'

It was a Monday morning and Ramya was my first client of the day. I hadn't even had a cup of tea yet. This was the first time I was meeting her, and I wasn't ready to be confronted with the cross-questioning, lawyer-style of therapy session yet. So, in response to her blunt question, I took a deep breath, smiled and held her gaze for some time.

'Do you mind breathing with me, please?' I eventually asked.

Ramya frowned. 'What do you mean? What's your answer? I need to know if you get me or not. I'm paying for your advice,' she said rudely.

In that simple yet agitated response, Ramya had given me cues to how defensive and guarded her nervous system was. She needed to test me in order to trust me. This was a woman fully in control of her experience. She was financially and physically stable, yet emotionally closed. My work had already begun.

'Ramya, I'm here with you now,' I responded. 'You don't have to decide whether I'm going to be your therapist or not, at least not so soon. You get to take your time—this is your process, a place for you and only you. I definitely won't lecture you on any basics of sex and sexuality if you don't need that. Many people assume that therapy is a space where the therapist doles out advice, but that is far from what I'm interested in. I'm interested in you, and your experiences. Now, please breathe with me and tell me, when was the last time *you* truly hugged someone?'

I'd offered Ramya a direct yet simple challenge by accepting her mistrust yet keeping the focus on her. Her irritation and defences were soon to be my responsibility to hold with her, as they would show up in our therapeutic alliance until she chose to let me in. And the older we are, the longer it takes.

Ramya seemed to soften slowly as that session went on. She told me that I was the first Indian therapist she'd seen after cycling through many white therapists in the small American town she lived in. By the end of that session, she said she experienced a resonance that she had not felt before with therapists of other ethnicities and backgrounds. As time progressed, Ramya took small steps towards opening her wounds in my presence.

She revealed that she felt bad that although she was single, had access to many dating prospects and had no sexual inhibitions, the prospect of casual sex solely for the sake of physical pleasure felt completely unattractive to her. She said that her friends could not understand her inner life, because most of them had partners or were married with kids. Ramya felt closer to her university students than she did to her friends or to her parents, all of whom seemed to be living in a reality completely different from hers.

Ramya confessed to being envious of the ease with which her friends accepted their status-quo and felt bad that she was a 'difficult person' due to her unique ideals. She wanted to feel at ease. Her friends, in turn, were envious of her ability to shift her life around according to her whims and fancies and often advised her to be grateful for her freer circumstances. 'But gratitude does not make me feel less alone, right?' she said.

One session, as we were exploring how Ramya had always chosen to stand by her ideals ever since she was a teenager, I asked her if she had ever considered herself to be queer.

At first Ramya looked taken aback and said, 'No, I like my men. Are you saying I should try dating women?'

'I'm saying there are many definitions of queerhood—some which go beyond defining queerness purely through the lens of gender and sexuality.'

I introduced to her the concept of 'neuro-queerness', first birthed into mainstream psychology by Professor Walker in their book *Neuroqueer Heresies*. Simply put, 'neuroqueer' is a term for anyone who actively subverts one's own cultural conditioning and one's ingrained normative habits and patterns to make space for a life that feels more authentic to them. They make decisions that put them further in alignment with their unique capacities, gifts, aspirations and hopes rather than following a path that normative socialization expects of us all.

So, a person like Ramya, who chose to dedicate her youth to an academic life first instead of forcefitting herself into the sociocultural expectation of having marriage and children for the *sake* of them, could also be considered an act of neuro-queerness. Ratna, Mr J's wife in Chapter 2, who chose to understand and accept her husband's closeted queer identity and then maintained her friendship with him, could be considered neuro-queer too. Mr J and her both subverted the rather popular narrative that marriages automatically and always break when certain secrets are kept. They invested in their relationship through choosing inner work practices together, prevented an ugly breakup and allowed their former marital bond to change into an aromantic, friendly, familial connection.

Ramya warmed up to this concept quickly and came back the next session having done a lot of research on this term. She started identifying with this label and even introduced it to her students. We laughed at her tendency to dive deep into topics that she liked, and then I expanded my offering. I said, 'Have you considered that although these labels help in making people who make non-normative choices feel more seen—and give us permission to celebrate that—they are limited in their capacity to do much else?'

'Tell me more,' she said.

I explained to her that people who follow the timelines that their culture and society deem normal also experience many social rewards for those choices.

An Indian woman who is married by the age of twenty-five and has had two children by the time she is thirty may not have a PhD. But by the time she is forty, she has school events to go to, college futures to plan for and extended family gatherings to host. Her social life tends to be full, whether she wants it that way or not. Queer people—and specifically queer women—who identify with this label tend to have no such social rewards. This is exactly what Ramya was experiencing.

As discussed in Chapter 2, this is why a lot of queer people choose to remain closeted and emotionally repressed. Coming out is not only an act of courage for oneself but also stands in courageous opposition to the milestones that mainstream society rewards as 'normal'. Ramya was experiencing tremendous isolation due to a lack of community of people who had made similar life choices as her. On top of that she was living in a racial reality that was far from her own, in a place where being brown and being tenured in academia was a rare combination.

All these factors made for an explosive mix for skin hunger, which is a concept that is very rarely discussed among us urban Indians. Skin hunger, which is also known as touch deprivation, is real. When you first chance upon this term, you might mistakenly think that this is a concept about the lack of sexual touch in someone's life. And when most Indians think about sex, it's about penis-in-vagina sex. However, sex and sexuality are much broader than that. The question of exactly what defines sexual activity is not clear cut and can vary between partners. Two hands touching can be as sexual or erotic for the partners involved as two penises touching.

Similarly, the deprivation of human touch that human beings feel is far more encompassing than just a lack of penetrative sex. Humans have a need for affirmation, protection, validation, acceptance, belonging and companionship even beyond or outside of sex. Touch is one sense that provides this to us viscerally. Touch is not only about sex. Think about it like this: India is an overpopulated country, where our public spaces are extremely crowded. In general, we don't really need to think about touch here as a valid need because we get it in our society every day—with or without our consent. In every public space in India—buses, trains and the street—there is always a lot of human contact. In our society, we have to find ways to not be overstimulated by touch. Yet, we feel its lack when it isn't present.

Indians sometimes complain about the lack of sensory stimulation in the West. The lack of colour, taste, smell, sound and touch feels apparent in a country that isn't as populated and whose aesthetic might not be as stimulatory. So, for many urban Indians, when this sensory need goes unmet, it can lead to feelings of emotional aloneness, of a lack of belonging and a lack of true connection with other human beings.

For Ramya, this was manifesting as feelings of isolation, a slightly desperate anxiety of feeling abandoned and a gnawing sadness about 'not feeling safe'. It was understandable that she did not desire casual sex at this time, for it felt to her like a rather inefficient substitute for her primal need of a heart-centred connection.

In 2020, the COVID-19 pandemic had created an avalanche of therapy demand. In 2019, I was receiving ten to fifteen queries a week for therapy appointments from people living in India. The next two years saw my office receive close to three hundred emails daily. I would say three-fourths of these appointments dealt with the issue of urban isolation. Before the pandemic, people who lived by themselves would retreat to their homes after spending all day in contact with others. When forced to stay at home all day, their homes started feeling sterile, even suffocating, because external stimulation had been removed. There was no one to retreat from.

Touch is a real need, and we all have tolerance levels towards it. In his book *The 5 Love Languages: The Secret to Love that Lasts*, author Gary Chapman describes how people interpret and express love in one of five ways: gifts, quality time, physical touch, acts of service and words of affirmation. People who have an affinity for the love language of physical touch tend to feel alone in relationships where they aren't able to express or receive physical affection.

Such individuals enjoy hugs and often give longer ones, even to acquaintances. They tend to enjoy giving and receiving massages, and like sitting close to other people. Feeling heard, seen and felt at a physical level is important for people who value touch the most, such as Ramya. These are the people who are at the biggest risk of suffering from touch deprivation.

In urban Indian society, women have more opportunities to access their touch needs through caring for their friends' babies or holding the hands of their platonic friends. Unfortunately, for Indian men—and cis-men in general— this need is severely stigmatized. Within patriarchal (meaning male-centric) societies that dominate many parts of today's India, patriarchal norms dictate how things are done. These norms are what create psychological conditioning, as discussed earlier. The roles of each individual tend to be predefined as rigid rules to follow, and deviation from these rules brings a large amount of pushback in terms of teasing, bullying, shaming and even social ostracization.

Although we may preach concepts such as gender equality on social media, it is still rare even in 2024 to find Indian fathers nursing babies by themselves. Men participating in activities that are considered traditionally 'feminine'—such as cooking, childcare and household cleaning—still causes social disruption. This imbalance transfers into emotional, sexual and psychological behaviour patterns too.

For example, men who express their feelings through crying are often judged as 'too feminine'. The conventional North Indian question *'ladki jaise royega?'*— (You'll cry like a girl?) which is offered as well-intentioned motivation in that culture when a man is feeling sad—is indicative of this reality for men. But this adage devalues not only how women are taught to express grief, but also shames crying—which is a natural, healthy form of emotional expression.

In smaller Indian cities, especially those that are less urbanized, it is a common sight to see two cis-men walking while holding hands platonically. In larger Indian society, holding the hand of a friend of the same gender identity isn't necessarily perceived as a romantic or sexual gesture but rather as a sign of friendship and camaraderie.

However, can you imagine two cis-men in an elite area of a major Indian city holding hands while going to work? This is a rare sight and would be quickly judged negatively as homoerotic and 'weird'.

By the time Ramya ended her therapy work with me, she had started accepting her skin hunger needs with less shame. She had understood that what she was seeking deep down was more heart-centred mental and emotional understanding, friendship and companionship to feel safer in her body, heart, spirit and mind. Ramya started to give herself permission to seek this both romantically on dating apps and platonically at work and hobby classes. She formed her own version of a family where she lived—a chosen group of people with whom she organized activities such as festivals, movie nights, book discussions and nature walks.

Ramya told me that she had benefited from expanding her definition of what a sexually mature life looked like. She trusted me a lot more towards the end than she had in the beginning and said that she would return to her inner work when she felt ready to do more unlearning about her judgemental stance and biases about others. Among these was harbouring negative judgement towards people who had less sex than her. She would label them as going through a 'dry spell'. I bid her goodbye and turned inwards to reflect on this term myself.

The term 'dry spell' implies that everyone's idea of a normal, sexually healthy life should include consistent sexual experiences that 'water' one's metaphorical sexual fields. However, not everyone views their sexualities as fields that need constant watering to be internally satisfied. People on the asexuality spectrum teach us this very important truth. There are people who are non-judgemental of their own sexuality and of other's sexual preferences and lifestyles. They may choose to have sex rarely, or only under specific circumstances, while being fulfilled and happy. Other people need consistent sex in their relationship to feel fulfilled—maybe once a day or few times a week—and it's something they manage with their partner's drives and needs. This is sex positive too.

I personally find the criteria for today's sex positivity definitions highly superficial. The quantity of sex that one has does not define how sex-positive and trauma-informed one is. One can be completely uninhibited sexually and still enact harmful stereotypes and shaming judgements on one's partners, friends and family. I believe that as long as you are not consciously withdrawing sex as a form of 'punishment' or as a result of deeper unresolved anger or shame—or shaming someone else for wanting more sex than you— then the 'sex positive label' applies to you regardless of how many times you yourself engage in the physical act of sex.

The mainstream discussion of sex positivity—especially among younger generations of urban Indians—brings with it an idea that if it is not sexually promiscuous, it is not sex-positive enough. This needs to be deconstructed. It is a harmful stereotype that shames people whose touch needs are not related to physical sexual acts.

So many of my clients approach sex-focused therapy as a type of confessional. Some have concerns about not having experienced sex by a certain age: 'I am thirty and I still haven't had sex! I'm such a late bloomer, please fix me.' Others, whose sexualities have shifted or they are experiencing a low libido, may say: 'I feel so ashamed I can't penetrate my partner. Isn't sex the main reason people get married?' I sigh deeply when people bring these self-shaming stereotypes to my desk.

I feel compassion for the burdens we carry as our own. There are so many diverse permutations and combinations to live as sex-positive, shame-free human beings who respect each other's authentic lived reality. And so many of these ways have nothing to do with how often you choose to create sexual pleasure with someone.

## Chapter Takeaways

Physical touch and emotional connection are fundamental human needs which are repressed in our urban Indian city lives and their lack can cause touch deprivation, isolation and loneliness. While being sex-positive is a good antidote, the concept of sex-positivity requires deeper thought in our cultural context. A sexually healthy society needs to be able to name, feel and work through one's shame around needing touch.

## Exercise 12: *Practise self-intimacy*

Here are some ways to remedy touch deprivation and deepen intimacy with yourself, especially if you're living alone, away from trusted loved ones:

- Touch trees and animals as often as you can.
- Take social media breaks and disconnect often. Once for thirty minutes daily can be extremely helpful too.
- Take slow, long, mindful showers where you spend time soaping each part of your body gently and practise being present with your body.
- Massage your feet, chest and genitals with an oil of your choice before you go to sleep. Touching our own body with mindfulness can relax stressed muscles and bring a sense of connection back to ourselves.
- Consider either adopting or fostering animals if you can. If you live in a country like India where there is an abundance of

animals living unattended on the streets, try making friends with a stray dog or a cat in your neighbourhood.

- Visit this animal often and stroke its fur with intention. The oxytocin released in this relationship can be an antidote to skin hunger for both of you.

- Read more books, listen to podcasts and watch talks by people who advocate cultivating slowness in the middle of everyday tasks.

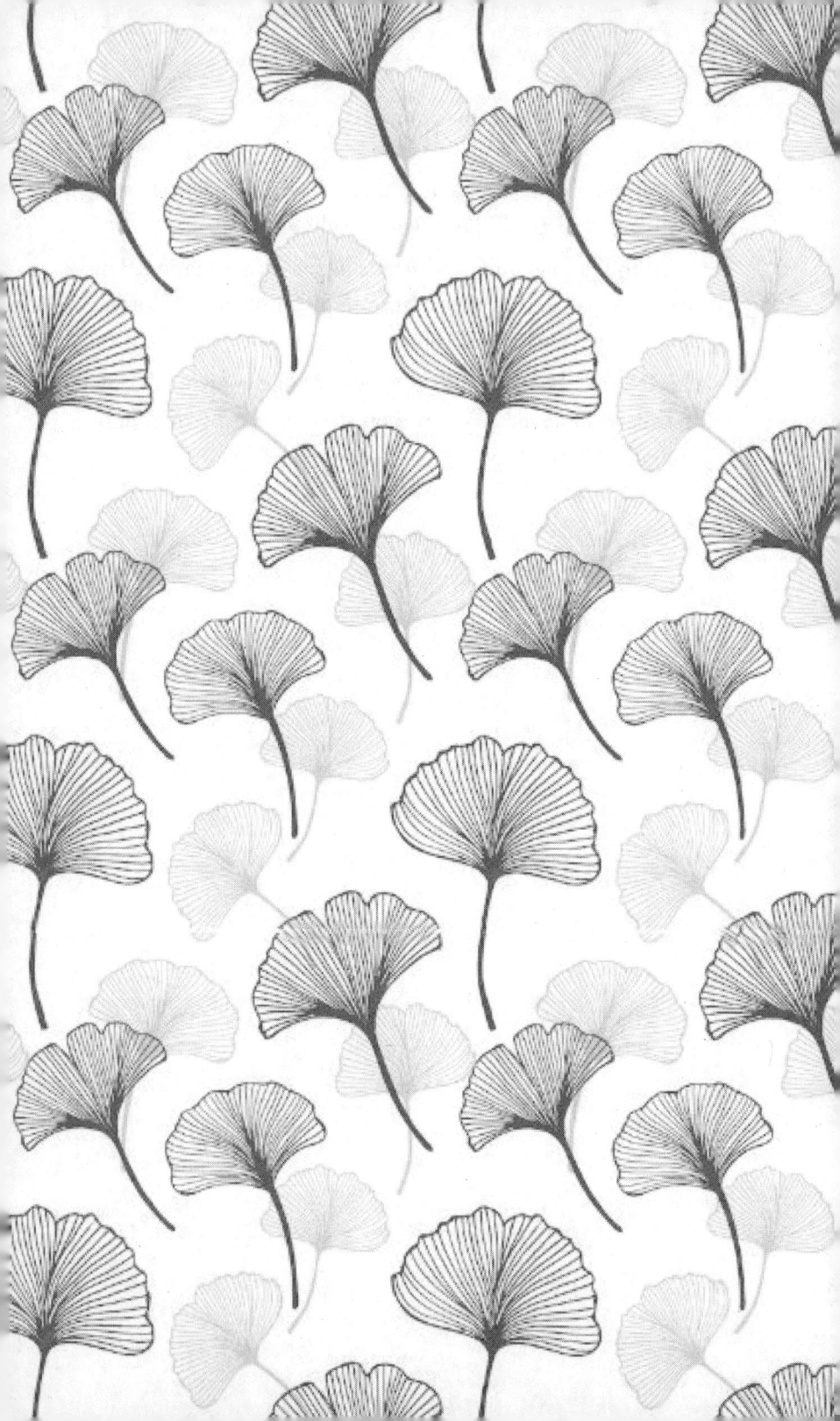

# PART 4

# Heal

### *How do we heal shame?*

*'Anything we love can be saved, for everything we love
emerges from the gentle flower of self-blessing.'*
—Alice Walker, author

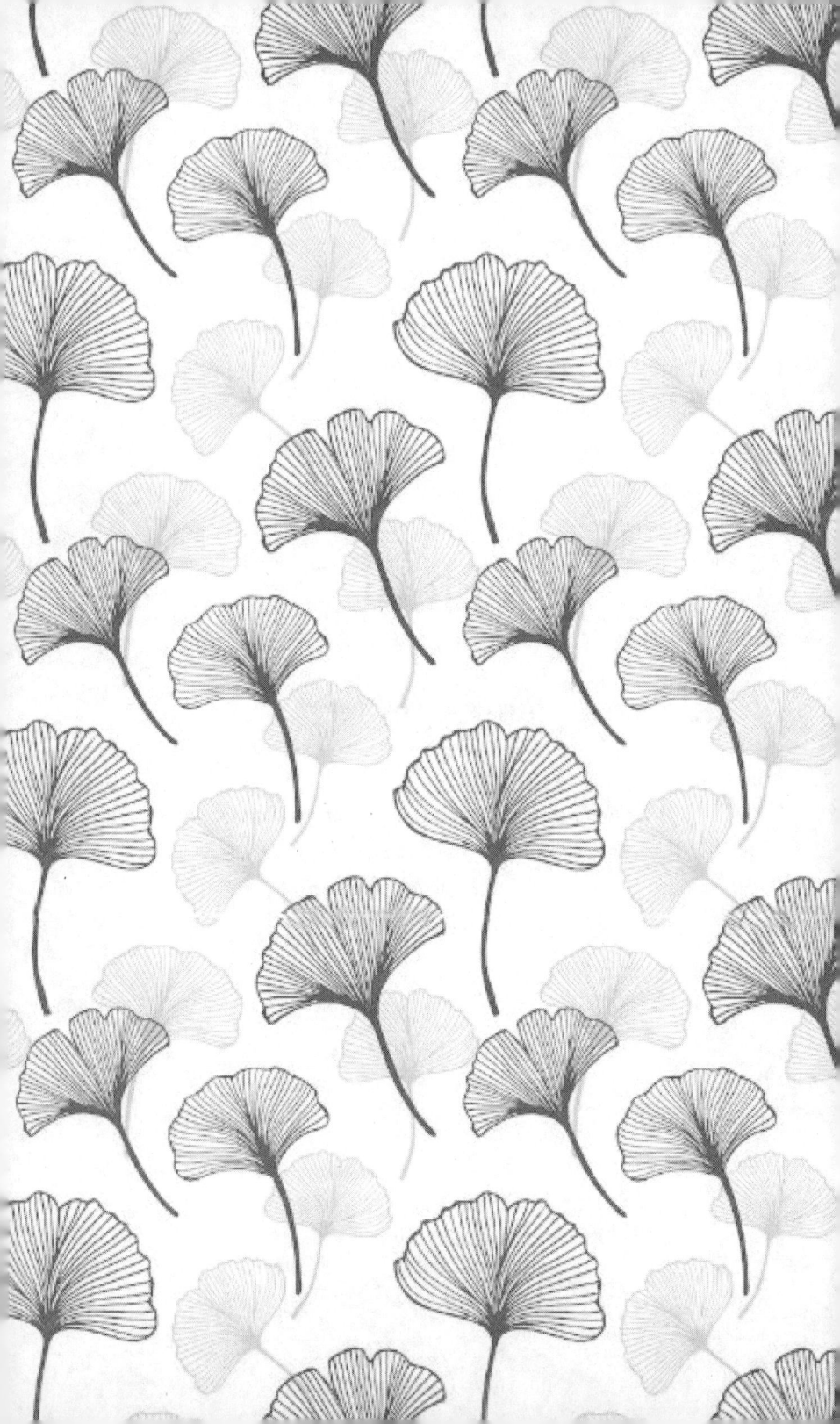

# CHAPTER 8

# 'You're not "broken" even if someone said you were ...'

## *On challenging painful narratives from the past*

It was in a drama therapy training workshop in 2009 that I first learned that clitoral erections existed. Those erotic-charged feelings of longing that vulva owners (anyone who has a vulva) sometimes experience in the morning were actually forms of 'erections'—clitoral erections to be precise. The participants of this workshop were asked to describe what desire and longing meant to each of us. After each person shared their thoughts in a group discussion, the facilitators talked about the science of clitoral erections to throw light on how female desire has remained shrouded in mystery. Due to patriarchal norms dominating the world for such a long time, these feelings of sexual stimulation—which are natural, biological, hormonal and even mundane—have not really been legitimized for vulva owners.

Just like men experience erections, so do women—and any other gender identity as well—in their own, unique way. In Biology class at school, I had learnt that the word 'erection' when it came to human bodies was solely used to describe what happens to penises when they feel aroused. I was also subtly taught that erections and penises were 'dirty'—these words meant something harmful and that I should always be alert about them. Penis erections have been demonized even for penis owners. The celebrated psychotherapist Esther Perel, often speaks about how as a society, we stop touching our male children after they hit puberty. She attributes this to be one of the main causes of deep, unresolved feelings of isolation and alienation, specifically in cis-men which results in many unhappy adult marriages and lonely human beings.

After gaining knowledge about clitoral erections in that enlightening, safe space of the drama therapy workshop, I remember wanting to discuss this exciting new revelation with all my extended group of university friends. It was also the year that I had chosen to come out as bisexual to a small group of friends, and the news had spread through college like wildfire. The popular insult going around about people like me at the time was that people like me were 'loose' of character, 'attention-hungry', 'broken and damaged' in character, in relationship to society's moral values, which, according to the people doling out these insults, was the only reason someone would study human sex and sexuality.

Years later, when I was living in the United States of America, in what is considered to be a more 'progressive society', I attempted to start a coffee table conversation on these topics with a married couple friend. My friend enthusiastically chimed in about her interests in the field, only to be labelled a 'hypersexual slut' by her partner at that time. He believed that it was too bold of us to talk about such things so openly and quickly dismissed much of what we did professionally as nonsense.

Needless to say, our friendship quickly dissolved after that ignorant attack. Both in India and in the United States, I have personally and professionally faced tremendous judgement for openly talking about topics that are considered taboo.

## Inner work helps subvert painful narratives

While these hackneyed insults that were flung at me did sting at the time, they also taught me a good bit about narratives, and the importance of subverting the harmful ones whose only purpose is to keep the receiver of those narratives hurting.

My experiences have taught me that shining light on what's buried brings up other people's shame. Some people would rather choose insults, attacks and lose cherished relationships in their lives, rather than deal with their own discomfort.

When people use insults to express their feelings, they're often reflecting their own psychological state. When we start to understand how much human beings project what they believe to be true onto others and create stories about other people based on their own experiences, we realize how much of a disservice we do to ourselves by believing people's shaming insults as true. Shame is a fascinating emotion to look at closely, and healing shame allows us the liberation of not taking on other people's negative projections as your own truth.

It is easy to emotionally react to people's judgements at face value and easier yet, to believe that they are saying something that might be true about you. But it is harder to confront the judgement, sit with it and try and observe its origins. This inner work, although uncomfortable, can be very liberating. Once you allow yourself to feel the sting of the judgements and the labels instead of turning away from them, you practise discerning your truth from the many falsehoods that are projected onto you. When we look at the phrases 'hypersexual slut', 'broken, damaged lady', 'homosexual sissy boy', 'weird loner', 'fat, intense auntie' or any such aggressive abuse more closely, we start to see how these labels speak more about the person who is doing the labelling rather than the person being labelled.

## What exactly is shame? How does it show up in our sexual health?

People think shame is just one bad feeling that we feel—just like guilt, jealousy, greed or envy. We often put all of these in one big box labelled 'negative emotions'. When asked to define it, most of my clients cannot really give this feeling specific words or even locate exact sensations in their bodies to make this emotion tangible.

We tell ourselves that the secret to a happy life is avoiding this 'negative emotions box' as much as possible and focusing on positive emotions. And we extend this binary way of thinking to the act of healing. We think that to heal is to remove, delete, erase, move on and avoid the negative. In urban India—a land filled with many methods, organizations and styles of inner work—the mainstream understanding of working on oneself through spirituality also gets reduced to fit the same binary view of good versus bad.

But deep down, our experience of reality is far more complex than that. With maturity, we realize that very few things in life fit the simple boxes of positive and negative emotion. However, our Indian social language keeps people stuck to old, outdated views and leads to shame persisting as a concept. Psychotherapists define shame as a mix of many emotions that have not been processed. Shame succeeds by keeping people stuck in old narratives, some of which you may have explored in the post-chapter reflective exercises.

When you want to control someone, the easiest way to do so is to bring up the part of their lives that you know they feel the most ashamed about and use it to hurt them. Shaming people is a horrible way of getting them to respect you or listen to you, but it works precisely because shame as a mixed emotion is a powerful concoction that stems from our core fears. It can be imagined as a complex, large, heavy enmeshed mix of feelings, stories, triggers, core beliefs and unmet needs that lives in our nervous system.

If I had to imagine my shame as I write this, it would be a big, red, amoeba-like blob that sits somewhere between my heart and my lungs. It is a place where I am currently also sitting with some grief at present. I know how my body responds to shame, and what exactly shame does to my nervous system. Through my own therapy and inner work experiences over two decades, I now have tools and pathways to access it, locate it and gaze at it—and, on good days, when I'm feeling internally resourced, to even confront it and ask it what it wants of me.

I just wonder how much internalized, unprocessed shame the people who used those aggressive insults towards me had about their own sexuality, their own bodies and their own natural curiosities. As you're reading this, does a similar shaming insult used for you come to mind? Have you experienced being sexually shamed? Have you ever shamed someone?

## Shame is a protective mechanism

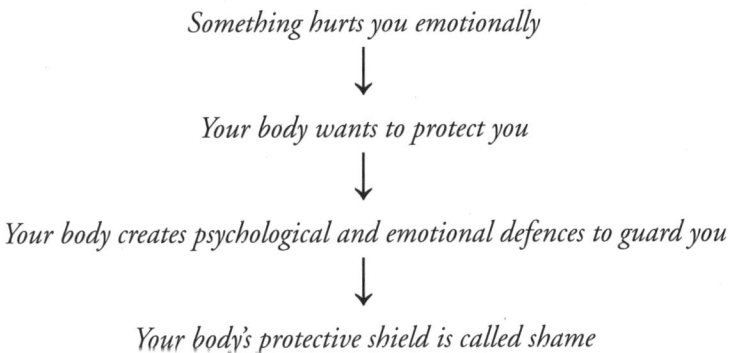

*Something hurts you emotionally*

↓

*Your body wants to protect you*

↓

*Your body creates psychological and emotional defences to guard you*

↓

*Your body's protective shield is called shame*

Like the conflict styles (fight, flight, freeze and fawn) discussed in Chapter 3, shame is often people's survival response. It is a type of defence mechanism. Underneath shame lies some form of hurt.

Think of it as a shield, or as a guardian soldier trying to protect a vulnerable child's bedroom from attack. Shame protects people from threat—and when we feel threatened, we're often feeling scared.

No one escapes the knife of trauma, but not all trauma is disruptive. Sometimes trauma shows up quietly in waves and cycles in relationships, daily life and families, impacting us in ways we never really understand. It is common human behaviour to not pay attention to feelings that make us feel heavy or bad. However, as you may have already gathered from this book, it is the exploration of that 'bad' feeling that leads us to insight. Insight is basically a deeper understanding that comes from our own explorations—not because we read a theoretical explanation about it or watched a video of someone explaining it. Insights often then lead us to an action step.

It might be useful to think of shame—especially sexual shame—as a heavy, large entity protecting or preserving some part of your body, mind, heart or spirit that has experienced some form of hurt. Most times, this entity called 'shame' does not listen to logic or to rational explanations why it should not exist—instead, it thinks it is doing its job by being hyper-protective of you. And many times, it ends up 'protecting' you even from the very things you might so deeply want—love, care, affection, understanding, sex, emotionally available partners, a supportive friend who knows your flaws and, most importantly, a loving relationship with your own self.

## How shame may have helped you at some point in your life

If we think of shame as a rock blocking your access to a lush forest, then we also could consider that maybe this same rock that we're trying to get rid of was possibly helpful at some point in the past. Who put this rock here in the first place and why? Think about Kusha, whose case you read about in Chapter 1, and how she discovered that her shame was a protective response against the childhood assault she faced. What comes to mind? Could it be possible that at some point the forest that we want to access wasn't as lush? Perhaps it was thorny, dry and full of predators—and that rock was there to help us stay safe.

Sometimes, children have to create protective mechanisms for themselves when nobody else is around to provide protection from external threats. Shame helps us to survive in environments we don't like and have trouble adapting to. We could be stuck in these environments without having any say in the matter. A home with difficult parents who didn't or couldn't fully see their children or who outright abused and continue to abuse them is an example of a dysfunctional environment filled with threat.

As discussed before, shame is a painful, mixed emotion which our body can utilize as a defence mechanism to protect us from abuse. As we grow older, we may have enough privilege to choose the environments we stay in. However, workplaces can also be threatening environments. If we are placed under toxic bosses who constantly put us down, we may have to learn to become defensive and keep our guards up. A client once said his boss—who would shame him for making small spelling errors in front of the entire office—was just like his abusive father. This client had unconsciously created a defence mechanism of people-pleasing behaviour to keep himself safe and would submit to his boss's abuse just as he had to his father's.

This client had internalized the shaming belief that he was a 'broken idiot who could not deliver perfect results'. Hence he spent his weeks at work doing everything his boss asked of him only to go home and have panic attacks about being stuck in this toxic workplace even though his skills and talents could take him somewhere better. The shame that was once protective was now causing harm to him by preventing him from taking action that would benefit him.

Do you know in which part of your body you tend to feel your shame? Locate where you feel fear, and your shame will likely show up in that same area. For many people, shame shows up as a hot, heavy sensation of anxiety around their chest. For others, it lies somewhere near the stomach area. Where in your body is it located at this moment, if you had to give it some attention? Now, let's look at what we do when we feel shame show up. Just like conflict, each of us has a different relationship to this feeling that varies based on our life experiences until now.

### Actions we take when we feel shame

Here's what some of my clients have told me about what they do when they feel shame:

- **'When I feel shame, I eat a ton of comfort food.** I'll find myself ordering at least two burgers and chaat and dessert. I may not even be hungry and might even have food in the fridge, but it just feels good to fill myself up. When I do this, it makes my bad feelings go away for that night. Of course, the next morning I find that same shame is back where it was, but at least my stomach feels bloated enough for my mind to focus on that instead of trying to work out my feelings.'

- **'When I feel that feeling that makes me believe that "I am bad, I am not worth it, I am just always going to be stuck where I am",** I start watching porn mindlessly. I seek more and more stimulating versions of porn and I know the more I browse, the nastier my porn preferences become. I know that I'm not actually horny and that I just want to escape my big, bad feelings and zone out for some time. But the difficulty is that "some time" becomes two hours, then three, then five. The next day, I wake up feeling worse about myself and guilty that all I did the previous night was numb myself without intention or true pleasure.'

- 'When I feel shame, I tend to want to drink or smoke a lot. When I first started going overboard with recreational substances, I didn't know I was doing it to soothe my loneliness. But now I know I drink and smoke so much not because I'm having fun, but because I just want to shut down those feelings I don't like. They remind me of how terribly broken I am.'

- 'When I feel shame, I tend to overwork myself. In some ways, my shame makes me want to punish myself. I start taking up extra projects at work even when my plate is already full. I think somewhere I believe that work will distract me so much that those feelings I don't want to sit with will go away on their own. They rarely do, though.'

- 'When I feel shame, I use dating apps like a zombie. I swipe left and right like it is a video game and chat with dozens of people, many of whom I'm not even attracted to. The moment they start telling me about their lives, I start feeling bored and distance myself from them. All my friends normalize this as the "dating scene". I start to feel desperate to have casual sex because I don't like being alone when I'm feeling these sensations of shame.'

- 'When I feel shame, I attack the person asking me to do something differently—even if it is a loved one or a therapist who I know has good intentions for me. I insult them for wanting to "fix me", I say something like, "Anyway, you are not good enough for me, so leave me alone. What do you know?" After this, I tend to want to be alone and I insult myself. I start thinking that I am so ugly and if only I had a larger penis, or larger breasts, a thinner stomach, or longer hair, a sexier smile and so on, I would feel less bad about myself.'

## How shame shows up in relationships as a defence mechanism

- 'When I feel shame, I try to run away from my triggers. Sometimes I know it is something my partner said casually that triggered me or made me feel ashamed, and sometimes it is an acquaintance's comment. At that moment when I'm feeling shame, my partner often tells me that I'm unapproachable and attacking towards him. I don't want to talk it out even when he begs me to. I dissociate and zone out of the conversation that is making me feel bad. I feel the need to get out of where I am because I feel terrible. My shame tells me I am not good enough for this person I like. My partner tells me I make it very hard for him when I do this.'

- 'When I feel ashamed, I start feeling small. I start thinking that my voice isn't very valuable. I find myself in relationships with partners who take up a lot of space and who need me to do a lot of work for them. The last partner I dated told me he loved me after two meetings. I got so swept away by his charisma, I moved in with him after only three weeks together. It was only after that did I slowly start experiencing his intense anger outbursts. I had somehow not noticed that he was rude, insensitive and didn't do much for himself. But I cooked, cleaned and held our relationship together for years. I think deep down I long for someone to love me back the way I overextend myself for them. I then catch myself thinking, "I'm not that great anyway, why would someone emotionally healthy want to date me? If I just become whoever my partner needs me to become, they'll think I am worth loving." One of my core beliefs about myself is that I can't say no because I know that person wants me to say yes. I need to agree to be liked and loved. I also believe that if I say no, they will think I am bad.'

- 'When I feel bad about who I am, I want to stay hidden. During those times, on dating apps I somehow match with people who are emotionally unavailable or married and being dishonest with their partners. I realize that my shame wants me to stay small and believe that I am unworthy of being seen, especially in romantic love.'

- 'My shame shows up as my saviourism. Deep down, I only feel worthy if I can be of use to someone. So, I start taking on everyone else's problems as my own, wanting to fix them or change them. I "work on" my relationship like it's an exam we both must pass. How come we are always fighting? Relationships should feel good a lot of the time. I don't want to feel this shame anymore.'

- 'When I start feeling shame, I start catastrophizing that people will find out that I'm actually good for nothing—just like my mother, father, sister, bully, teacher or guru used to tell me. I jump straight to the worst-case scenario. I think that I am not worth it and that I am "bad", so what is the point of trying if I am going to fail anyway? Those people who originally said that about me may actually have known me better than I know myself. These are some thought patterns that repeat when I feel ashamed.'

After a few sessions of inner work and therapy, many people say they had no idea that these externally chaotic behaviours had any link to their internal experience. I remember an extremely honest therapy session during which a client and I had unpacked their body dysphoria and shame-based gluttony. That session had been challenging and intense and had opened up some deep vulnerabilities in my client, who was emotionally avoidant. I half expected them to want to quit therapy after that.

To my pleasant surprise, they said, 'It is such a relief to understand the roots of my shame. I thought there was no logical reason for me to do this and, perhaps, I was just very broken, damaged, lazy and unchangeable. But since I've become more aware of how my body works, I know that these behaviours are like shame spirals and I can see myself reaching out towards them when I'm upset. It is liberating to know that I can do something about this feeling of feeling broken.'

Instead of teaching people how to navigate the very normal and healthy aspects of our human sexualities, we make erotic desire and adult play seem cheap and dirty. There is a lot of cultural shame associated within our landscape for desiring consensual touch and play as adults. Clients tell me that they are unable to express these longings in any part of their mundane lives for fear of being judged as 'perverted' or worse, 'sex-obsessed'. Hence, any kind of 'safe space', with a trusted family member, a non-judgemental friend or a therapist or a life coach feels like much awaited relief.

Shame is one of our defence mechanisms that keeps us protected from truths we don't want to, aren't able to or aren't ready yet to see. Defensiveness shuts down negative as well as positive input from the outside and keeps us believing in our present realities as the status quo. When we dislike the feeling that shame gives us because our mind is judging it as negative, even threatening, our bodies naturally want to stop that feeling. This is why when someone who has been very defensive and closed off for many years is asked to reflect on something they said or did, they experience that invitation to lower their guard as threatening.

We saw in the chapter on intergenerational conflict that families which remain in defensive mode around each other most of the time likely feel very ashamed of themselves deep down, whether they admit it or not. When someone is very defensive, it can be expected that they will want to hurt whoever tries to breach their defence because their nervous system is perceiving them as a threat. They become dishonest and lose connection with themselves.

The unfortunate consequence of remaining highly defensive and stuck with shame-based feelings, beliefs and thoughts is that one also misses out on taking good risks. If we miss out on reframing the idea of being 'broken', we cut ourselves off from meeting new, open-minded people, from our creativity, from learning to repair conflict and experience deeper relationships and from the joys of therapy and expansive inner work—things which lead to an abundant life.

## We heal shame by tending to its wounds

We heal shame by challenging the narratives it leaves us with, in playful yet courageous ways. We heal shame by not internalizing the shame that society projects onto us. Our parents model conformity to the oppressive parts of our culture's socialization instead of showing us that things can be different and that each family can pick and choose what works for them based on their own needs. Most of us carry this heavy burden of other people's shame for decades, complaining about its weight and how bad it feels inside us, without realizing how we've also taken that untruth as our own truth. It is not our job to do so.

All humans are on some part of the sexuality spectrum and we all need this part of our identity validated, affirmed and supported in whatever way we feel comfortable. Trauma healing happens when we understand that there is nothing 'fundamentally wrong' with any of us. None of us are 'broken' or 'damaged' from the inside. Healing happens when we internalize the truths of our bodies' ways and learn that our big, bad feelings are pathways of expression for our bodies that point towards what may be hurting inside us. Trauma healing takes place when we see that many of our problems are in relationship to social systems and psychological conditioning that doesn't fit the evolution of our minds, hearts, bodies and spirits.

Many external behaviours are responses to inner realities, history and patterns. What hurts us is the rigid socialization of living in 'rape culture', following fixed gender rules while being policed, being taught to believe the myth that one race is superior to another and that one body type is more deserving of attention and love than another. They keep us stuck in shame. Being trauma-informed, going to therapy and learning about our parents' trauma is often mistaken for blaming one's trauma history. You have perhaps heard the remark that therapy is a way to blame one's mother for all of one's own problems. However, this is a sad, misguided notion of inner work.

Trauma healing gives us access to inner power, which then allows us to melt our defences, including shame. It is our authentic power that gives us the motivation to shape our futures in the way we deem fit. A trauma-informed approach to existence sees every human being as a unique amalgamation of responses to various causes and effects. They are shaped by nature and nurture but also by their behaviours and hopes. We must remember that every person has access to resilience and choice.

To heal shame, we have to go towards it. You have to *work on* shame as if it were an ice-block or a rock—you can't work against it by ignoring or avoiding it. When we melt our shame, we automatically melt our defenses. With melted defenses, we experience the breaking away of stagnation and, eventually, forward movement.

While this is hard work, with persistence the rock breaks down into pebbles that you can store away in your pocket as you see the forest more clearly. With time and consistent efforts, inner work becomes joyful, pleasurable and nourishing. You are not 'broken' even if someone said you are. Please utilize the exercises in the following section of the book to deepen your access to your own power.

## Chapter Takeaways

All human beings belong to some part of the sexuality spectrum and we all need this part of our life experience validated, affirmed and supported in whatever way we feel comfortable. Trauma healing happens when we understand that there is nothing 'fundamentally wrong' with any of us. None of us are 'broken' or 'damaged' from the inside. Understanding the nuances of how shame can make us believe differently is an important milestone of the healing journey.

## Exercise 13: **Unlearn shame-based narratives**

This exercise helps to make deeper internal connections for yourself. This is a private, intimate exercise, for your eyes only. So please create space for yourself to explore this question if you are open to it.

*Think of a time when you were under the age of ten and were exploring your body for pleasure. Perhaps you were playing with parts of your body in whatever way felt playful to you, finding its shape and turns or experiencing its newness—until someone interrupted that process, in either a positive or a negative way. Perhaps a parent found you exploring, or maybe a family member about your age. It could also have been the doorbell that interrupted you.*

*Think back to whatever your experience was. What do you remember being told to you? Are there any rules, any embarrassing feelings, any constricting sensations or unpleasant memories surfacing?*

- Write about this experience in your journal.
- Now, complete this statement:
- *When I was a child, I remember feeling embarrassed about _____ in my body.*
- Write as many answers that come to mind.

.................................................................................................................

.................................................................................................................

.................................................................................................................

.................................................................................................................

.................................................................................................................

.................................................................................................................

.................................................................................................................

.................................................................................................................

.................................................................................................................

.................................................................................................................

You've just named your first memory of forming a narrative around exploration, body and play. Now, think about the following deeply:

- Consider the situation you were in—were you in a public place, where an adult gently and kindly stopped you without shaming you, and redirected you towards appropriate self-touch?

- Or was it when you were in your bedroom, and an adult invaded your personal exploration with anger, blame and projections of shame onto you, like in Kusha's life?

- Or was it when you were in school, and the teacher or other authority figure punished you by humiliating you in front of your friends for something you did not know you were doing with your body? Like in Rahul's life?

Consider taking some moments for reflection towards these questions. If you feel the need to draw, paint or write about it, feel free to do so. As you engage in this exercise of sexual storytelling for your own mind's eye, material that you weren't aware of might come to your attention. If you're working with a therapist, consider this topic for your next session. But for now, reflect on the connection between your earliest memory of being told 'no' about your body, and your own narratives around self-permission.

What comes up for you?

Could it be that our sexual triggers, cultural conditioning, sexual defences, moralities, desires, kinks and more could be encoded in an embodied map of sorts? Do we all carry this map with us wherever we go? And if we do, could it then be that this very map also has the solution to the things we struggle with?

When we allow ourselves to be curious about our own challenges, kinks, queerness, psychological defences and needs, then that curiosity can sometimes lend us the power of self-compassion. Imagine a world where we felt so empowered by the acceptance of our own complex maps that we automatically felt it was natural to try and accept someone else's.

The more different someone's map might be from us, the more curiosity this self-acceptance could give us to lean into the challenge of learning what triggers that person or shuts that person down sexually, mentally, emotionally or physically. Our cultural codes are currently breaking and, with them, crumbles the metaphorical wall of silence in India—the wall that blocked the voices of survivors of sexual violence, of marginalized populations of our country and of queer people who were told their sexualities were 'broken' for being different from the norm. When walls break, certain social defences crumble and a lot of repressed material rises to the surface of social consciousness.

When people who don't often speak the truth confront the truth in themselves, they're often left shaking and anxious after speaking. We might think the shaking, the panic and the anxiety is all because of the power of the acceptance of this truth itself, when the reality could be that those responses are our body's way of telling us that we are distressed because we have not been confronting this truth all these years.

The path then clears for deeper truth-telling because bodies often function best when there is minimal internal psychological conflict and resistance. Bodies don't want to carry burdens. One of the greatest gifts of true inner work is to understand how to use the power of our own healing gaze to accept our internal conflicts.

# CHAPTER 9

# 'You get to craft your own path forward.'

*On breaking the cycles of intergenerational sexual trauma*

Each time a mother teaches her daughter about taking care of her sexual health, about expecting mutuality in relationships, about standing against interpersonal violence or about leaving abusive relationships, she gifts her daughter a lifetime of messages that impact the quality of the daughter's life. When a father educates his son about the menstrual cycle after the son reaches puberty, about releasing his anger through exercise, about saying sorry to his wife in front of his children and meaning it, he creates decades of inner stability that the son will be able to lean on internally when life's challenges come his way.

Now consider the opposite. When parents are actively violent towards each other and refuse to resolve conflict in an emotionally healthy manner, or when they make insensitive and crude comments about people different from them, they're indirectly passing on those same values and ways of viewing the world to their children. When these children grow up, they often find themselves in relationships with similar patterns, behaviours and worldviews.

The six-year-old watching his father slap his mother may become a twenty-three-year-old who doesn't know how to control his impulses when he is in conflict with their partner. The ten-year-old who took on the role of 'mummy's best friend' is now an over-functioning forty-year-old who can't see herself outside of her caretaking tendencies. Adult children might be exhausted and even chronically ill from never having learnt to say no, but they might continue because this is what they thought was 'normal' for the first decade of their life.

## Intergenerational trauma is real

At fifty-one, Kusum had been through three long-term relationships, all of which had ended with her cheating on her partners. She had been to astrologers, gurus, coaches and therapists in an effort to understand why she couldn't break her pattern of sabotaging her relationships. When she eventually consulted with me, I suggested she read Mark Wolynn's popular book *It Didn't Start With You*. The book's main message was that trauma isn't solely an individual problem, as the field of psychopathology has opined, but it is a type of wounding that can last for generations as feelings, sensations and genetic stress responses that can get passed on from one family member to the next. This is what is defined as intergenerational trauma. Even though a person didn't personally experience a particular type of trauma in their lifetime, they could be feeling its symptoms because their grandparents experienced a more severe form of it. The book explains the value of tracing one's family line in connecting the dots to find out what could be carried forward.

The trauma of race and racism is passed on generationally and there is ample new research available on this, especially in the United States. The trauma of colonial oppression, religious displacement and oppression and caste-based oppression have similar narratives in India. When people are not given the opportunity to heal from trauma, they're likely to live in a state of distress. This can lead to a range of negative outcomes for themselves and their descendants.

## Intergenerational relating is hard

Their children may experience difficulties with attachment, disconnection from their extended families and culture and high levels of stress. This in turn can create developmental issues for the children, as we are particularly susceptible to distress at a young age. It creates a cycle of trauma in which the impact is passed from one generation to the next. Now, add to this the unique Indian familial setup of many generations staying together, or at least somewhat close together, and we have intergenerational trauma compounded with relational challenges, in a fast changing social landscape, all butting heads simultaneously.

For Kusum, this sparked interest in her exploring the relationship and marital patterns of her parents, grandparents and great-grandparents. At first, when she started asking her family members these intimate questions, she came across shame, embarrassment and judgement—and interestingly, a lot of secrets, mixed narratives and silence as well.

Persisting, Kusum discovered a series of abandoned marriages on her father's side. Three generations of the men on her father's side had married young and then suddenly left home around the age of thirty, leaving their wives and children behind without support. Kusum was flabbergasted when she realized that her first long-term relationship ended at thirty-one when she cheated on her partner with her coworker. While her family's chronic history of relationship sabotage is no excuse for Kusum's own infidelity, the knowledge that she wasn't broken or alone in this pattern helped her greatly.

Intergenerational patterns have been studied quite deeply in children of alcohol addicts and smokers. The evidence-based research in the field is continually evolving and filling the vast gaps in knowledge that still exist. As mentioned earlier, verbal dialogue about intimate trauma histories is not a welcome language in our culture. Colonial trauma has been barely understood, even though Independence was over seventy-five years ago. Caste-based trauma narratives are often dismissed as invalid and irrelevant in mainstream upper and middle-class urban India. Thus, many of us are only starting to understand how our histories are not mere stories of the past that can be just put in a box and erased, but that ancestral legacies continue to live inside of us. This is precisely why open discussions on uncomfortable social truths are so important at this stage of our society.

Although there is an abundance of wisdom alluding to the concept of intergenerational trauma patterns and ancestral healing in many parts of Hindu folklore and scripture, the disconnection from them in the English-educated urban Indian mind is deep. Also, there hasn't been enough work done yet in translating this indigenous knowledge into contemporary academia to allow greater understanding and contextualization of this knowledge within the fields of Indian and international psychological research and practice.

Young urban Indians are often given many messages of 'breaking free from the past', as if the past is one big dirty stain that needs to be eradicated for the appearance of a fresh, new 'blank slate' from which we will suddenly start to lead more authentic, sex-positive lives. I've seen innumerable advertisements, films and well-meaning sex-positive communities that follow this rather superficial narrative. While it's valid to question older ideas and knowledge systems, our past does not suddenly just disappear if we apply the ethos of 'cancel culture' to it. As the concept of inherited trauma proves, the past gets carried forward into the present, which if left unexamined, shapes the future accordingly.

During my personal yoga practise, I find myself surprised by moments of stillness in which I see parts of my body moving in ways that my mother's or my father's body moves. A certain pointedness of my ankle, a certain bend of the shoulder and a quiet sigh reminds me how much the people whom we're genetically linked to live inside of us, whether we like it or not.

Varun, a twenty-five-year-old pilot, lived with his fifty-five-year-old father, Vijay, in Dubai. Varun's mother had passed away when he was young, and he was his father's sole support system. Living in Dubai for work meant being away from his dad, so Varun had recently helped Vijay migrate from Kerala to Dubai to live with him. After his father moved in with him, Varun faced a major struggle to share space with Vijay after years of living alone.

Varun was dating a woman from a different religious background. They were also sexually active and were considering moving in together. His father approved of the partnership but disapproved of their intimacy. He expected Varun to remain celibate until marriage. He would often fat-shame Varun and crack misogynistic jokes, which would be off-putting to both Varun and his partner. However, Varun would say nothing. Acting from his 'flight' trauma response, he failed to set active boundaries with his father in a way that the parent could understand.

Due to these value differences, Varun was finding it extremely difficult to share space with his father. Our therapy work focused on finding ways through which this family could have better ways of navigating their life together. Varun was an avid reader and proponent of mental health awareness and followed all the popular psychology social media accounts for tips and tricks to make his life easier. Unfortunately, each time he tried to apply a popular social media therapist's advice on setting boundaries with his father, their relationship would turn even more hostile and aggressive. It led to them not talking to each other for weeks while living in the same apartment. Slowly, the situation was devolving into them considering two separate apartments, with different kitchens and different house helpers to make their coexistence smoother.

## Intergenerational bonds are our cultural strength, and need to be navigated sensitively

It is important to remember that a lot of mainstream psychology information is written by and caters to white people living in white-dominant cultures. Mainstream healing content is not written for and by brown people for our unique contexts. It has been written by EuroAmerican practitioners for their contexts and then the rest of the world is expected to adjust to it. City dwelling, English-speaking, more westernized urban Indians instantly adapt to this Western-generated content because it makes sense to us intellectually. Yet, it is more impractical than helpful for us.

When he came into therapy with me, Varun said he appreciated one of my social-media posts in which I had argued that it was illogical to apply Western-focused ideas of what a good boundary is onto more relational, community-focused cultures like India. This is where I see the pain and disconnect in this boundary language and its practical application in urban India. We try to make our families understand words like 'boundaries' and 'triggers' but they don't resonate. Boundaries are not isolated words that can be simply honoured outside our specific context. As we engage in this difficult process of growth, we have to be mindful of all the ways our specific cultural context suffers from its lack of visibility. Asian cultures are more relationally inclined and the punishments for breaking these relational nets are severe— caste oppression, social ostracization and financial dysregulation, among others are some examples of these punishments. Hence, some of the examples of 'healthy' boundaries in Western cultures are seen as very rude and selfish in other cultures.

While boundaries are an internal concept, the way boundaries are received depend a lot on how they are communicated. Healthy boundaries for one family system might look entirely different for another. If we use cut-and-dried boundaries in urban India, we may get more pushback than we expect and then have to deal with the strong reactions to us setting such boundaries. Decolonial therapy is about making concepts appropriate for context.

Blanket statements such as 'healthy' or 'unhealthy' ways of relating to each other don't apply in India. What was considered healthy for an older generation of Indian parents is extremely different from what's considered healthy for their children, especially because of the rapid economic, social and psychological shifts that our country has experienced since Independence. We are presently at an extremely polarized point in our shapeshifting society, and we will need to think of innovative and diverse ways to solve the oppositions we're seeing in our homes and at our workplaces.

## Therapy as an aid to intergenerational relating

When atleast one family member is open to change, family therapy sessions can melt years of opposition caused by communication challenges amplified by unaddressed problems. When there is a large amount of resistance and suspicion towards revealing private problems to a third party, like a therapist, a notion that is common in our cultural context, I suggest individual therapy to the family member who is the most willing. This strategy helps the individual member of a distressed unit gain the skills needed to begin to de-escalate conflict, which is often much awaited progress for the family. Slowly, in due time, some of the deeper challenges such as irreconcilable value differences, differing lifestyle needs and more are then addressed.

On the subject of contrasting values and shared space, a rather unique anecdote comes to mind. Every year, I try to make a trip to the Himalayas. I find it to be a pristine place for contemplative inner work. There is a spot in the Parvati Valley that can only be reached by a seven-hour uphill trek. Even for women who like travelling solo, it's perhaps best to take a friend since it is a rather inaccessible point. It is one of those rare places where time seems to stand still. Here, the mountains melt into the river, the river becomes the forest, the forest expands into the mountains, and before you know it, you're sweating in freezing snow at the edge of a cliff.

Interestingly, in a place like this our bodies have a magical way of forgetting the boundaries between elements. This place reminds me of a time where I shared personal space with a friend who had values dissimilar from mine. I lived in the Parvati Valley with him for ten days as neither of us had been able to convince any of our closer friends and family to join us.

Through our conversation, it was clear to us both that we didn't particularly take to each other's personalities. We just did not understand each other as we differed in political views, in ways of making sense of the world and even in our basic sensitivities of what was around us. Yet, somehow we were intrigued by each other's unfamiliar ways and hence decided to travel together to this place—a place sacred to us both but for totally different reasons. We could not agree about anything, but we could not stop talking about the fact that we did not agree. It was an eccentric friendship.

And so, during our arduous journey together—interspersed with hours of silence and individual meaning-making—we just came to accept that we disagreed completely. Our polarization lived by forming a compartment of its own as we moved together—then separately, then together again—from mountain sludge to slippery rock. Somehow, we accepted that we didn't have to align fully to coexist, to breathe and to drink in the beauty around us. And, most importantly, we did not have to agree with each other to respect each other.

Years later, we continue to revisit that strange trip that gave us insight into this unique acceptance of each other as travellers on dissimilar paths depending on each other for logistical security. In a fantastic way, that time shaped us both into who we have become today. We are not friends, but neither are we enemies. He returns to my inbox when he wants to share a new insight about that trip, and I do the same. And that's where our contact ends.

In this non-normative connection, there is a true lesson that I often revisit. It's especially relevant during times like these in which many truths are finding it hard to coexist due to a lack of justice, of patience, and of listening to each other. There seems to be a need for us to find comfort in exactly similar viewpoints, without which we find it hard to respect or even accept people and their individual differences. The mountains share such insightful lessons in interdependence, if only we listened.

## To connect with loved ones across generations, practise active listening and good boundary setting

During a therapy session with Varun, I shared the anecdote about my trip to the Parvati Valley with my unusual companion. I tried to help Varun see that the polarization he was experiencing was impacting both his fathers' and his nervous systems, making them more inflexible and closed off to each other. I asked Varun if he had tried listening, validating and making his father feel understood first, and then telling him clearly what Varun would like him to do differently. 'Have you asked him why he wants you to remain celibate?' I asked. 'Have you told him that it hurts your feelings when he calls you fat? Have you expressed to him that if he continues you'll have to keep conversations short with him?'

We were at a crucial point in our therapeutic alliance, where Varun needed to challenge his internalized shame and move beyond the narratives of victimhood he had decided were his norm. Instead of ending the session by telling Varun how unfortunate he was to have a father who talks in shaming insults and how sad I was for him, I had put the onus back on Varun. This was a push against Varun's identification with his helplessness, and he seemed shocked at my suggestions. He left my office in an unsettled state of contemplation.

## To connect with a loved one across generations, don't over-nourish shame

Indian socialization is an emotionally driven one. When people feel blamed and shamed here—especially as older adults—they tend to split into childlike states of emotional immaturity. This state often renders them unable to hear multiple perspectives or to sit with their children's lived experiences. The only solution to avoid psychological splitting is doing inner work. While we can wait for all the generations of our family to reach a point of inner maturity from where they can access therapy and inner work, the reality is that that could take lifetimes to happen. Not everyone in one's own family is or will be open to seeing their part in dysfunctions, nor will they always be open to changing it.

Because many Indian adults live with their parents and other older and younger adults, the responsibility of learning how to communicate with one's family in ways that they can understand falls on the shoulders of the one who is growth-oriented. This can be experienced as burdensome by the growth-oriented person and they can view themselves as the eternally sacrificial 'victim'.

This is the story of almost every Indian household, and many Indian adults seem to wish for a more emotionally available set of parents who can share the emotional labour of the family in a fair way. Unlike in Western countries, it is not a practical possibility for most Indians who have differences with their families to move out and reduce everyday contact with them. Our culture is highly enmeshed and doing so can even become counterproductive. While the ideal situation is to have family arrangements like Bindu, Rajeev and Ninaben do—where each person can have their own space and can choose the quantity and quality of their intergenerational connection—this is not financially possible for most of us. This can keep a lot of people stuck in the narrative that they are victims of their parents' emotional unavailability, way into adulthood.

When I ask you to challenge the narrative of victimhood, I want to make it clear that I am not implying the existence of victimization itself. Victimization is a debilitating process that can make us completely lost, hurt, destabilized and helpless. Victims of intergenerational trauma often have their lives completely shaken up by what happened to them, and dismissing victimization entirely would be utterly insensitive. However, there is a difference between suffering victimization due to traumatic events in one's life and choosing to always prioritize the narrative of one's inner victimhood.

## To connect with a loved one across generations, listen with your heart

In Indian family systems, heart-centred emotion-based communication works better than the dry, and rather blunt style of communication popularized in the West by social media. People of Vijay's age have been conditioned by their parents that children must have emotional and physical proximity to their parents and families. For them, the word 'boundary' is perceived as threatening—because it signifies a wall, and a wall signifies distance.

Thus, many Indian parents of an older generation feel attacked when their adult children ask for their valid needs to be met. They hear 'setting boundaries' as 'my child wants to leave me'. Varun experienced some cognitive dissonance upon hearing what I was asking of him. He saw himself very much as the 'victim' of his dad's insults and lack of understanding and respect. He did not fathom that he also had agency to shape the way he would like this relationship to go.

The following week, when Varun returned to therapy, he seemed eager to share. 'No, I haven't really taken the time to listen to why my dad believes what he believes,' he told me. 'I thought that by doing that he'll think it's okay to talk to me the way he does. In fact, now that I've had time to think about it, I think I might be bulldozing him with my wants and expecting him to read my mind. Even if I don't agree with him, perhaps I need to be able to tell him that I am old enough to make up my mind about my sexual choices and maybe also assure him that I'm not abandoning him for thinking differently from me.' I was thrilled with Varun's insights on this matter. From that session onwards, Varun actively worked on learning to speak his mind with less shame and personalization.

# To connect with a loved one across generations, learn to de-personalize

To feel fully but not become the emotion is one of the most difficult skills I teach within psychotherapy. When we personalize, we see the world happening not just around us but *to* us—and not just to us, but *because* of us. We internalize the events we encounter—words, actions, developments, problems—and magnify our role in them. We take on not just the event itself but the *causality* of that event, often believing that we are responsible for how it went down—especially when that event is negative.

In many ways, personalization is a form of *self*-blame. It takes our emotional response to an event and turns it inward so that we become the primary mover. The emotional effect of personalization can vary, but it usually involves some common sensations: stress, anxiety, depression, burnout and a sense of extreme responsibility coupled, ironically, with powerlessness.

Personalization is just one of several so-called *cognitive distortions*—exaggerated or irrational beliefs that cause us to perceive reality inaccurately. In other words, personalization is a function of ego. This isn't inherently good or bad. It's just a feature of our species. Our egos—or our identities—can't *not* take things personally, because they experience *everything* personally. We can only experience life *as ourselves*, so everything that happens, by necessity, happens *to us*.

When we over-nourish the parts of ourselves that were or have been victimized and choose to lead all conversations with it, this can sometimes make our domestic life experiences more difficult. Choosing to navigate the world through our own victimized parts is a way of telling ourselves that the only way to live in this world—to get one's needs met, to be heard, to be loved, to be understood—is through the language of pain. People can then get very attached to this pain, and see themselves as stuck inside of it, rather than being able to exercise agency and personal power. These concepts are explored in a deeper way in the following chapters.

I like to think of our psyche as a wild forest filled with plants of many different varieties, all of which need a different kind of nurturing. When we keep watering the plants of our victimization, let's say, we end up nurturing only that part of our inner forests, at the cost of drying up everything else. This results in harbouring mental patterns which have learnt to thrive only on pain. One day, when something new tries to grow, it suddenly has no space in our psyche. This new plant may need a different kind of watering. It may need us to learn new ways of nurturing it, perhaps in a new direction, maybe it needs us to keep it in the light a bit more. It needs us to work with it differently. But we get to stuck in pre-decided roles and narratives, that it becomes hard for us to sustain this new growth.

Please remember that no individual adult can play the same role their entire lives. No mother can only remain in the role of a mother and no father can only remain in the role of a father all their life. If we ask ourselves if we have been able to play the same role all our adult lives, we might realize that we haven't—that it's not possible to do it. It is one of the most heartbreaking yet liberating things to understand (and herein lies our own access to our power) that people play different roles all through their lives. Whether they play those roles well or not is a separate (but important) matter.

Adults play many roles, and those roles often transition and move around in our interconnected lives without us being able to 'see' this clearly and slowly. I love psychotherapist Sheldon B. Kapp's nuanced work on this subject, that he writes about in his existential

psychotherapy book, *If You Meet the Buddha on the Road, Kill Him!*.
He describes in-depth the liberation that awaits every adult, beyond
the phase of trauma victimhood, where one realizes that one has
an intrinsic power to drop old roles and craft one's own life path
forward. The interesting part about the power of agency, he writes
profoundly, is that accepting this—however long it may take us to
do so—helps us not only own our power, but to give **other** adults
agency as well. When Varun started setting boundaries with his
father with gentle assertiveness and compassion, he and his father
made way for a new kind of relationship and a more balanced way
of relating to each other's difference. Varun had stopped putting his
father up on a pedestal and started seeing him as his own flawed
yet loving human being who needed to be taught how to connect
to his adult son. His father, after the initial bumps that come
with new boundaries, had learnt to perceive his son as his adult
human being with a set of values that were unique to him. This
acceptance helped both of them embrace their own personhood
better, instead of submitting to their hitherto self-sacrificial roles as
the norm. The debilitating relational conflict stopped entirely once
this foundational relational challenge was met, and their days were
marked with the occasional, harmless familial spat that is common
in any long-term relationship.

## Chapter Takeaways

Trauma isn't solely an individual problem, but is also a type of
wounding that can last for generations of family systems as feelings,
sensations and genetic stress responses that get passed on from one
family member to the next. This is called intergenerational trauma,
and shows itself in relationships. Earlier, within the Indian cultural
context, relating intergenerationally was considered commonplace.

In an increasingly individualistic society, intergenerational conflicts are increasing and the ability to co-exist, decreasing leading to a tendency towards greater personalization of emotional pain and rising conflict. Practicing active listening, depersonalization and learning to reframe unhelpful narratives can be effective ways of relating across generations more smoothly.

## Exercise 14: Practise expressing difficult feelings to people you love

Let's walk through how to express disappointment, annoyance, irritation, anger or hurt to your loved ones in ways that will improve the chances of you getting heard by them.

Let's consider the example of a mean comment. Consider that your father commented on your weight in front of other family members, which made you feel ashamed and angry at him. You felt triggered. You understand that may not have meant malicious harm towards you, but instead of not saying anything and resenting him, you would like for him to know that his comments were hurtful. How will you communicate your anger with compassion and assertiveness?

## Step 1: Feel your own uncomfortable feelings fully

When there are uncomfortable emotions involved, it's tempting to skip the first step itself and launch into any of your trauma responses - fight/flight/freeze or fawn. Instead, first practise feeling the charge of your emotions fully without acting on them. If you feel a trigger arise, pause what you're doing and let your feelings take their course in your body. For instance, if you're at the dinner table or at a holiday gathering and feel a big emotion arise when a family member shames you, take a deep breath, stop talking and utilize the pause to allow the feelings to move through your body.

You might have any or all of the following thoughts:

'I feel really triggered.'

'I want to fight this out.'

'I am so angry—how did this person say such a thing about me?'

If you've ever tried feeling your reactionary feelings fully, you might know that this takes some practise. Our reptilian brain's reaction is to keep us outside of threat, so we tend to jump to a highly personalized reaction because we tend to feel threatened by what we disagree with or feel attacked by.

## Step 2: Make sense of your story for yourself first

Now that you've paused, contemplate: what is hurting me about this comment and why?

As you start to think about this, your mind may offer you a few explanations. Allow the stories in your mind to form. Freewrite some of them below.

For example: When my father, or mother, made xyz comment about my weight, I felt bad because:

...........................................................................................................................

...........................................................................................................................

...........................................................................................................................

...........................................................................................................................

...........................................................................................................................

...........................................................................................................................

...........................................................................................................................

..................................................................................................

..................................................................................................

..................................................................................................

..................................................................................................

..................................................................................................

..................................................................................................

..................................................................................................

..................................................................................................

..................................................................................................

Once you complete this, you'll start to understand why you felt so hurt. Your triggers from the past may surface. Perhaps your father made similar comments 3-4 times in the past when you were feeling most vulnerable, or maybe he can sometimes be a tad bit insensitive. You can now start to intellectually understand the impact the comments had on you. A story like this might start to emerge:

*I'm feeling really disappointed because I love my father and didn't expect this insensitivity from him. I guess I have an expectation from him that he is not meeting.*

## Step 3: Find the most sensible time to communicate this to the family member

(a) Now that the story is clearer, soften your heart towards them. Affirm the following in your mind:

*'I want to understand my father/mother and I want to be understood by him'.*

Self-affirmations can bring our guards down, and wire our subconscious mind to expect a positive outcome.

(b) Frame the conversation in a way that starts with the positive and then go towards what upset you in the moment. Here's an example:

'Papa, I remembered something you said the other day and felt myself getting hurt by it. Generally, I know you talk positively about me, so I thought you would know that I'm hurt by what you said. Do you mind telling me what you meant by xyz comment?'

Once this part is done, allow the receiver (your father in this case) to have his reaction to what you said. Remember, difficult conversations cannot go by script, but there can be a rough plan. The more practise you get, the easier these will become.

## Step 4: Now, let it go

You've done what you could and it's time to detach from the outcome of your work.

- Try belly breathing for ten seconds.
- Shake your body.
- Do a gentle neck rotation where you're sitting.
- Get up and walk around your chair.
- Drink a few sips of water.

Allow your body to take its natural time to move through these steps, don't rush through them.

## Exercise 15: **Reframe shame-based personalizations**

Personalization, as discussed in this chapter, is a *cognitive distortion*—an exaggerated or irrational belief that causes us to perceive reality inaccurately and makes us believe in our fears. This is an exercise that can help you 'flip the script' on some of the internalized shame-based narratives that you may be carrying within your psyche that have not been challenged.

1. Name the narrative:

   Perhaps there is a certain comment said about you in your family that triggers you each time it is said by a loved one, an insult that a family member doled out when you were younger, that shaped your self-belief so deep, that it would benefit from now being challenged. Think on these lines.

For example:

- *When I visit dadi/nani/ajji (grandmother), she says I seem lonely, it must mean she is scolding me for being so old and unmarried.*

- *Now, separate the comment part from your part of its personalization:*

   ....................................................................................................................

   ....................................................................................................................

   ....................................................................................................................

   ....................................................................................................................

   ....................................................................................................................

Using the example above:

Comment: Dadi said I seem lonely.

My personalization: I believe Dadi is scolding me for being so old and unmarried.

Comment:_____

My personalization: _____


2. *Now, challenge your personalization part:*

A few questions you could ask yourself:

- Is my personalization a reflection of the truth?
- Am I overgeneralizing based on something that happened in the past?
- What memory did the comment bring up for me?
- Did I feel powerless or out of control?
- Am I currently in my trauma responses (fight/flight/freeze/ fawn?)
- Am I personalizing my loved one's internalized shame/ insecurity about their own life?

3. *Now, write more of your personalizations down like the examples below:*

- If papa says I'm fat and look bad, to me it means I'm ugly.
- If papa says I'm fat and look bad, to me it means I'm disappointing him.
- If papa says I'm fat and look bad, to me it means he's not proud of me.

4. *Lastly connect the dots. Fill this table below using the example that is filled in:*

| What made me feel ashamed/angry/upset/disappointed? | Investigate your feelings | Include multiple possibilities about why your loved one said what they said | Reframe your thought |
|---|---|---|---|
| Describe the comment, the joke, the analogy or whatever it was that hurt you in as much detail as you can. | What felt bad to me about this comment?<br><br>What memory did it bring up for me?<br><br>Did I feel powerless or out of control?<br><br>Am I currently in my trauma responses (fight/flight/freeze/fawn?)<br><br>Am I personalizing my loved one's internalized shame/insecurity about their own life?<br><br>Am I overgeneralizing based on something that happened in the past? | Instead of focusing on the worst possibility that your loved one intentionally meant to hurt you, are there other reasons for why they said what they said? List them below | Modify any extreme 'splitting' language that has come up in the previous answers.<br><br>Replace it with gentler words.<br><br>Write down the more reasonable, reframed thought |

| Example: | | |
|---|---|---|
| I felt really bad when papa said I had put on weight in front of all our relatives. He always laughs at me loudly . Because of him, everyone chimed in. | I felt demeaned, and like I was the butt of the joke in the family. I am anyway so hard on myself about weight loss, could he not have been more sensitive? Am I so fat that my whole family needs to make fun of me? | Maybe papa thought I would take it lightly? Sometimes, papa doesn't understand how sensitive I am. | I felt sad that papa was not more sensitive towards me.<br><br>I feel sad when someone I love doesn't take care of my insecurities.<br><br>I may need to tell him this. |

Helpful questions to ask yourself in every conflict with someone who differs from you in your values:

- What role am I playing in the intergenerational conflict in my family?
- Where can I benefit from having more boundaries?
- Where can I benefit from being more accountable?
- Am I missing parts of the entire story? Have I dismissed my part in making this dialogue mutual and respectful?
- Have I expressed my values clearly?
- Can I tolerate my boundaries?
- Can I allow my family members to have their own reaction and opinion about what I am saying?

Please note: Reframing your subconscious and conscious beliefs is a powerful inner work exercise that can shift the nature of relationships. However, it yields the most powerful results when there isn't active abuse going on in the family or household. In case someone is actively abusing you and causing you harm intentionally on an ongoing basis, it would be prudent to first seek physical and emotional safety for yourself.

# CHAPTER 10

# 'Be brave, laugh, take it easy'

## *On antidotes to healing shame*

Do you remember those much-dreaded mandatory debate contests in school? How about those elocution competitions where each student had to speak on a pre-decided topic publicly at the school assembly as a way of practicing one's public speaking skills? If these do ring a bell in your memories, then you might also recall that the first couple of times one tried to use one's voice fully in front of a large group of people, most people experienced tremendous gushes of fear. In the school I went to, teams of students would rehearse their speeches for weeks, maybe months and yet, when it was time to get up on stage, each student's palms would become sweaty, our throats would start to constrict and we would stutter to find the right words. We would call this the '"shutting down" first time anxiety' phenomenon. It is a widely agreed upon notion that the anxiety experienced at the first attempt of trying anything new is often unparalleled. In terms of public speaking as a skill, it is only by the third or the fourth attempt in most cases, that one feels some degree of confidence in performing decently. And it is only by the twentieth attempt or after, once there has been a sufficient amount of practise, much trial and error and only after having become the butt of many jokes, that one can safely achieve mastery in truly speaking extempore with skill and charm simultaneously.

Similarly, it could be that the first time you choose to challenge your shame through choosing to speak up for yourself instead of staying quiet, you end up feeling worse than before. The first time we exercise agency to confront our repressed parts, those old patterns of fear can come rushing back, asking us to choose old habits.

## Courage is medicinal

This is where it is crucial to remember that one of the most direct antidotes to fear and shame is courage. Practicing inner work or therapy is like taking the rotten parts of a dried-up wound and applying lemon juice on it. It stings, but it's that very sting that breaks open the stubborn muck our nervous systems build up to keep us safe and numb. As you practise not shutting down every time the sting of your truth beckons, you heal. This is why things feel worse once you start inner work—before they start to feel better.

When we don't use the courageous parts of our inner voices, we condition our bodies to choose fear. And fear makes us believe that it is essentially 'bad' to tell our truths fully, stick to them, advocate for them and allow their wisdom to guide us. It attempts to convince us that if we did choose courage instead of fear, that choice might lead us to a ghastly outcome and we may be left abandoned, alone, desolate and hurt.

Truth-telling is one of the most direct antidotes to healing fear and shame. But truth-telling requires us to accept that other people, even those we hold near and dear, are not entitled to—and may not truly understand—the reasons and complexities of our truth. When we allow ourselves to remain okay even if someone disagrees with our truth-telling by trusting the inner ocean of security we've built through our inner work practices and insight, the heat of shame cools.

## Playfulness is medicinal

I define wellness as an internal process of becoming more at ease, more playful, more tender and more joyous in the face of life's inevitable calamities and contradictions.

We live in a fast, dense, emotionally and psychologically defensive world. Our guards are always up in these broken systems, our nervous systems seem trained to sense the next threat. Urban city life with its ever-increasing demands seems to be making it harder to access deep states of rest, relaxation and rejuvenation. This is not any one person's fault or responsibility but rather a function of the many broken systems modern life centers itself around. Jung in his book, *The Earth Has a Soul* holds nature in sharp contrast to the hypervigilance of modern existence. While he is certainly not the first inner work or mindfulness teacher to seek inspiration from nature's ways of seeing, he most definitely won't be the last. When I immerse myself in the wild forests, the salt beds, the coral reefs, the desert plains and the mountains of India, I find those spaces to be spiritually uplifting and emotionally nourishing. Instead of experiencing an energetic drain like most cities make my nervous system feel, I often return replenished. I find nature to be a rather chaotic teacher of multiple wisdoms.

Nature has many cycles, many answers and many processes. It can be healing but can also be violent. It isn't passive or lazy to embrace healing and wellness as an eternal process of sitting inside the depth of not knowing. We mustn't interpret the above as: 'I don't know anything anyway so I'll do whatever I want and life will take care of itself.' Not knowing is an active state in which we can challenge ourselves to go deeper within our own knowledge and find new answers even where we've looked before. The more knowledge and experience we accumulate, the more difficult it is to deepen one's life.

The nature of today's knowledge system, especially in healthcare, is to 'fixate' on a particular view, idea or methodology. However, it's truly liberating to me as a practitioner to stay connected to my practice of holding the wisdom of not knowing in one hand and the wisdom of knowing in the other. Practicing holding dualities and contradictions with greater ease has been one of the greatest pleasures of inner work for me. It often acts as an antidote to the social anxiety and collective trauma we are experiencing as a rapidly shifting cultural landscape.

## Slow down, it's okay to not know all your answers

Life is messy and unpredictable, and so are our bodies. As noted physician, Dr. Alex Comfort writes in his book *The Joy of Sex*, 'Religion and psychiatry have unfortunately misread the play-function of sex and sexuality and set about converting what nature programmed as turn-ons and resources into hangups. Playfulness, like tenderness, is something our culture has undersold.'

Playfulness, especially in intimacy, asks for the 'expert' to relax. We cannot play if the players are too focused on getting it right. We can play when there is flow in the game and when the players are focused on the actual task of playing—which by itself is a messy process full of twists, turns and chaos. Inner work is also about play.

When I chose to study art therapy over clinical psychiatry or allopathic medicine, I was following my intuitive voice—which was telling me to choose a profession that will allow me to make space for innovation within the craft of medicine. As a studious young person, I harboured limitless curiosity about human behaviour.

But try as I might, the textbooks and worksheets of conventional psychotherapy and psychology programmes seemed extremely dull to me. I was attracted to the arts.

When I was fifteen, I would often take my sketchbook out and doodle after hours of studying for my board exams. My mother would find me dancing to erratic beats on the radio or making music in my room even as I studied for the next day's exam—and she would say nothing. She always permitted me to create my own processes of absorbing mundane school textbook information. Her wisdom of leaning into her child's natural tendency towards play ensured that she did not cut me off from my own flow. Thanks to that, I now intentionally support people in crafting spaces for play in healing, both in my professional and personal life.

Play is a subtle entity and cannot be easily measured on a graph. So much of what is called 'inner work' is similarly subtle, as are the best forms of long-term intimacy. When we teach ourselves to embrace the wisdom in play, in intimacy and in healing, we also embrace the wisdom and the truth of the intangible. While a statement like this can sound esoteric, the fact remains that healing, at its very core, is a non-tangible process. It's not always visible and it isn't flashy—and there is no announcement when it happens. There are no numbers to prove how far one has come and no 'takeaways' at the end of every curve like in business.

Your friends and your lovers might not understand what you're doing, and this might feel difficult—especially when those perfectionistic cycles come back in the picture and ask for your attention. Your parents and your bosses might not perceive your inner movements. But most subtle work, when done consistently, leads to long-lasting changes. If you ask anyone who runs, writes, paints or cooks every day, they can attest to this unconditionally.

## Self-compassion is medicinal

So much of inner work lives in our ability to take pauses with our mental patterns even when everything externally may be going out of our control. You can find your trauma work living in yourself when you find that there is gentle allowance between light and shadow in your heart and you're stepping away from the intellectually heavy need to control either of those contradictions. Inner work is successful when you can taste quiet joy in deep connection with a lover, a friend or a family member. You can tell that your inner work is a living reality inside of you and has borne some fruit when you naturally find yourself one day choosing to relax into the anger about the same old thing that always used to rile you.

When you can feel your shame melting, your triggers softening, your voice becoming clearer, your heart opening and your mind allowing you to be messy and unfinished, you can tell that you're deepening in your understanding of life's challenging ways. Inner work leads you to quiet afternoon silences even in the company of family members who don't get you at all. When you use the tools of depersonalization, you arrive at the realization that shame thrives only when it is fuelled by belief in the abusive voice. Healing lies in pushing ourselves to deepen without getting lost in the chaos of our messy depths.

While inner work may not give you the most desired social recognition, it might align you to what truly brings you joy and long-lasting fulfillment. So much of inner work is a non-binary endeavour, which leads to a state of self-acceptance and contentment when you accept that not everyone will be able to understand your authenticity. And that is okay. The renowned psychologist Carl Jung describes reality as a beautiful prison of understanding and misunderstanding and says that in the centre of that non-duality is a joyful stillness of existence. Inner work is the opposite of today's fast social media culture—in which we learn to become impatient with our own processes if we don't understand something quickly.

Healing is an internal process of melting. It is natural to feel anxious when we start to see positive changes in ourselves. It speaks of deep motivation to maintain a state of wellness. However, instead of building a relationship with this anxiety with presence, play, joy, laughter, lightness, tenderness and gentleness, we are often taught to become strict, harsh and taskmaster-like with ourselves.

We can take on the voices of the very authority figures who caused our first experience of traumatizing shame and find ourselves saying, 'Look, this is not enough. You are not doing enough. Work harder. Are you going deep enough? Something is definitely going to go wrong with you if you don't. Before that happens, keep "working" to find fault with yourself so that you can use another tool to eradicate that fault.'

This narrative can quickly play into an endless cycle of fault finding with ourselves and our loved ones, because this goal of wanting to eradicate all faults within oneself is a perfectionist fantasy that is essentially anti-reality and anti-life. However, it's not at all your fault if you habitually slip into this, and the capacity to change this habit is inside of you. But the mainstream health and wellness industry don't want you to access this inner capacity. This industry profits off making people feel bad about who they are.

We aren't taught from childhood to transform our inner relationship to how we view our pain. If we were, we would have a less fragmented existence. Instead, we're taught to mentally split into either of two very chronic extremes: grin and bear your trauma or avoid, ignore and compartmentalize it. Wellness is about learning to transform one's inner abusive, shaming voice as well.

## Softening the inner critic

The harsh, critical inner voice that we can call the 'inner critic' simmers down. However, a curiously cyclical behaviour also takes over when we first start to heal. I often see it in clients who are new to the world of trauma awareness and healing.

This cycle needs to be nipped in the bud if you see it in yourself too, because it is counterproductive to the unpacking of shame. If allowed to remain, it can also stop new growth from happening. Simply put, the behaviour cycle goes something like this:

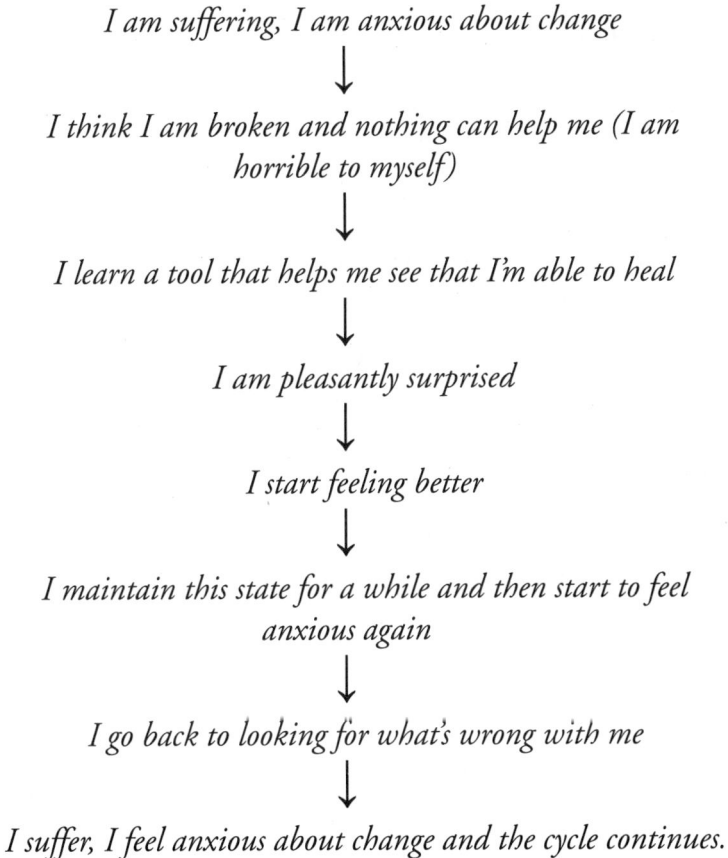

*I am suffering, I am anxious about change*

↓

*I think I am broken and nothing can help me (I am horrible to myself)*

↓

*I learn a tool that helps me see that I'm able to heal*

↓

*I am pleasantly surprised*

↓

*I start feeling better*

↓

*I maintain this state for a while and then start to feel anxious again*

↓

*I go back to looking for what's wrong with me*

↓

*I suffer, I feel anxious about change and the cycle continues.*

Often, when we discover inner work after years of living with our fear and shame, we can get extremely motivated to change and want to see results. We tend to become highly focused on the 'work' part of the process, keep analysing patterns in ourselves that we find concerning and bring them to light. In therapy, I do applaud my clients' conviction when they get to this point of the process, but it is also at this very point that I engage in teaching them to set boundaries with themselves. Sometimes, people can completely miss the fact that healing is not another task to perform on their way to becoming a 'flawless' version of themselves. Healing is not another form of self-delusion and self-abuse. This can take some time to understand.

## Chapter Takeaways

Performing small acts of courage even when you feel afraid, introducing spaces for creativity and playfulness in your everyday life and being gentle and compassionate with yourself are the three main antidotes to sexual trauma listed in this chapter. As you complete the penultimate chapter of this book, try resisting one-dimensional, simple answers to complex, non-binary concepts like the mind and our sexualities. Embrace those difficult sensations of shame, foster feelings of play and joy and try to soften that harsh inner critic.

## Exercise 16: Practise self-compassion

### The Mountains of Inner Stories Exercise

This is an exercise to soften our inner gaze and allow self-compassion to be internalized by ourselves.

- Bring a blank sheet of paper and a writing tool that feels pleasurable to you.
- According to this metaphor, you climb a mountain in each decade of your life. So, if you're thirty, draw three mountains on the paper. Draw more or fewer mountains if you're older or younger. Each mountain represents one decade and symbolizes the uphill battle that life can be. Growing older can be symbolized as having climbed many mountains.
- If you're halfway through a decade, you can find a creative way to represent half a mountain if you like. Don't worry about getting it right—this is an art exercise for you to play inside of.
- Now write the decades of your life down on each mountain. For example:

  Age 0–10: Mountain 1

  Age 10–20: Mountain 2

  Age 20–30: Mountain 3

  Think back to the decade for Mountain 1. What was happening in your life in this decade? What were some major positive themes? What were some difficulties?
- Choose an element from nature to represent this decade of your life. So, if you felt very open, warm and extroverted in your first decade, represent that with the image of a sun, a red flower or a mango.
- Continue this with all the decades of your life. You might start noticing that it was in the second decade that the sunny energy of your personality dulled. Or perhaps it was the opposite. You can use images such as a withered flower, a rotten fruit or a bigger, more fiery sun. Play with images, words and meanings for every mountain.

- Next, step back and see if you can pick out any patterns between the different decades of your life. See if you can tell how long the phase of you being like the sun lasted. At what point did you change into another element? Mark it on the mountain valley. As you take your time with this creative exercise, you'll start to see your life looking like a play of different colours, seasons, textures, themes and challenges.

- Lastly, close your eyes and try to allow yourself to feel the long, exhausting and adventure-filled growth journey your life has been. Visualize the sensation of having climbed a difficult peak. Imagine you're standing close to the edge of it, looking back in gratitude for yourself, your body, your mind and your spirit. Try saying to yourself, 'I thank myself for having come so far.'

However long and shapeless you think your growth journey is and however exhausting, hopeless and difficult you experience your process to be, the fact that you are engaging in inner work is a matter of pride. I hope you are proud of your efforts to step into greater self-awareness!

# CHAPTER 11

# 'Now that you know, keep at it.'

## On sustaining habits of change long-term

People often want to stop therapy and inner work as soon as they start to feel just a little bit better. We expect change to happen instantly from sporadic nudging here and there. We think it's okay to not go into the root causes of our pain and to keep swimming on the surface because it is easier to do that. But the reality is that long-term, sustainable change requires consistent work, which in turn requires patience. It is patience that gives us the power to sit through our contradictory, chaotic thoughts and feelings and transmute them into beneficial actions instead of harmful patterns.

Patience, however, cannot be magically created if we don't, at some level, enjoy the process that we're undertaking. This is why making space for joy and rest as integral parts of your trauma work journey becomes so crucial. Rest, laughter, humour, play and wonder—as described in previous chapters—are intangible in today's fast-paced, growth-oriented urban Indian society. These are easy to bypass as secondary. However, doing so would be making a crucial error and can set us up to become overwhelmed. We may burn out of the process of healing very quickly.

## To sustain change long-term, understand its stages:

Despite what romantic comedies like to portray, researchers studying human behaviour have proven that change happens in distinct stages and not in one drastic, explosive event. In the late 1970s, American researchers James Prochaska and Carlo DiClemente at the University of Rhode Island, developed the 'Stages of Change' model, which categorizes six stages a person goes through when they attempt a change in their behaviour.

- **Pre-contemplation**: I don't think I need to change. Everything is fine.
- **Contemplation**: I guess I can consider changing. Some things are not okay.
- **Preparation**: I'm reading up, analysing and planning for what I need to do to change.
- **Action**: I am putting my plans into action. I am performing the habits that will lead me to the change I want.
- **Maintenance:** I see some results and now I need to be consistent with my habits.
- **Relapse**: I am back to feeling like I did before I tried to change.

They defined change as a cyclical process, and human behavioural patterns moving back and forth between the different stages.

For a solution-focused therapist like me, the action stage feels very exciting. At this stage, I see one of my favourite new patterns of behaviour open for clients attempting radical healing. I like to term it the 'action step'—where one gains access to one's own inner power. It's a beautiful stage in which I've witnessed clients hold themselves accountable to the growth they choose for themselves without lies, excuses, shame, fear or victimized wounding. The energy of this behaviour pattern is contagious, and I leave sessions feeling empowered to attempt something difficult or new. Healing a wound without falling into the trap of getting stuck in the inner victim's voice leads to such a deep relaxation and ease inside of us that another internal 'door' opens automatically.

I don't have the exact scientific word to describe this gateway to someone with a more rational bent of mind, and you can disbelieve my lived experience if you so choose. However, since there is not much written about this, I'd like to name it here: this 'door' is the 'doorway of inner power'. Clients create art, music, dance and movement pieces, business plans, poems and even financial visions at this point because they tend to feel limitlessly creative and abundant. I can only define this in terms of feeling since my work lies in the realm of making feelings and sensations more tangible.

I have seen this doorway of inner power open in the advanced stages of trauma work in many of my own clients and I've experienced it in my own inner work practices, especially in the presence of teachers I admire. This is a space, a capacity or an ability that lives inside all human beings and helps to take their life path in their own hands and create it themselves. Despite many false starts, lost tangents and missteps over years of joyous labour, this creative potential eventually gets internalized during the healing process. That is when I know that my client is well on their way to living a fiercely unashamed existence.

## To sustain change long-term, practise emotional honesty with yourself on a regular basis:

I'm often asked questions such as: 'How do I trust myself more to access this inner power you speak of?'; 'How should I reduce the anxiety I feel about most things even after I melt my shame?'; and 'How do I make sure I won't fall off the bandwagon?'

My response to all these questions is: *emotional honesty*. It is a process of truth-telling with yourself and your loved ones that is gentle yet firm. In it, you keep your own promises and tenderly pick yourself up whenever you fall.

When you keep holding yourself—and please remember, the key here is your *own* self—accountable to the person you want to be, the life you want to shape and the relationships you want to have, you're sending your brain a message that you are trustworthy. You are playing a part in rewiring old shaming beliefs and replacing them with self-dependability. This builds strength in your internal self and gives it the capacity to hold its own when life throws more unexpected twists at you.

A healing self-accountability is a tender inner gaze that has the power of discernment. It is our wise inner guide who knows when we're picking that same old self-abusive pattern and shaming ourselves or others, and it knows when we're choosing new actions. For example, when you say you're going to do something, attempt to do it. Try your best. When you tell yourself you want to start a new habit or date a certain kind of person, take baby steps in that direction each day.

When it's hard to keep yourself away from whatever pattern you want to break, and yet you succeed in pausing your shame spirals

even briefly, you'll see your anxiety decrease significantly. If you change your mind about something you decided earlier, be honest and practise tender truth-telling by communicating that to those impacted by your choices, even if it's uncomfortable. Living in truth is a very scary but liberating, unashamed form of living. Living in truth doesn't mean telling everyone what you think of them or throwing your opinions of the world at everyone. But it does mean being truthful with yourself, and with others if they are willing to share the truth.

Society conditions us against this and against learning how to even feel what inner truths are. As described in detail in earlier chapters, urban Indian society teaches us to distract, numb, suppress, bypass, intellectualize and hide our innermost truths. It teaches us anything but how to feel our feelings fully and learn from them. When we try to achieve a state of 'feeling better', we forget that it's temporary. The human condition is like that: we feel better, then worse, then feel better again and the cycle repeats. When we stop expecting to 'feel better' as a permanent result and instead try to get better at riding each feeling as it comes without getting overwhelmed or throwing them at someone else, then we master the cycle of feelings. We then become okay letting them come and go as they need to, and we trust their inherent wisdom.

## To sustain change long-term, breathe deeply and trust your process!

Healing sustainably needs us to endure some amount of pain (not abuse), and one cannot know how much pain one can and should tolerate if one does not understand one's own sensations. Each person's capacity for pain and for change is different, and everyone has their own unique timeline according to what they perceive as important to them.

## Chapter Takeaways

Inner change is a slow, non-linear process that goes through stages. When one starts to make some progress, one can also jump ahead and stop inner work altogether. This would be unwise. Holding oneself accountable to some form of structure through a daily ritual such as journal writing can be a beneficial practice. Practicing emotional honesty and keeping promises to oneself can help in deepening one's capacity for insight and self-awareness over time.

## Exercise 17: **Write in your journal**

- Which chapter of the book did I find the most interesting? Why?

- Which chapter of the book did I find the least interesting? Why?

- Which was the chapter of the book that upset me the most? Why?

- Whose life story in the book did I connect to the most? Why?

- From having worked through the exercises in this book, what have I uncovered about myself that is the most difficult for me to accept right now?

- Have I become better at 'sitting with' my uncomfortable feelings, even by a small measure? (Refer back to Exercise 1 in Chapter 1)

- Is there a tangible action step I can put in place for myself to continue my inner work practice?

# Acknowledgements

One of my earliest spiritual teachers, philosopher Jiddu Krishnamurti considered the practices of listening and observing with total attention to be key to a liberated human existence. Shirdi Sai Baba, my ancestral spiritual guide, taught devotion and patience as pathways to heart-centred living. I feel grateful towards them for their influence on my life.

As I conclude this book, I find myself thinking, on a personal note, of a few things that bring me a sense of ease and closure at the end of each therapy day—the sweet aroma of the yellow champa (frangipani) flowers that decorate the windows of my office garden, the soft caresses of the kittens that live in it, the tight hugs that my clients give me when they leave for their adventures. All of these elements have lead to this book. I feel grateful towards my family, my parents, Sajani and Narayan, who nurtured me with devotion, to facilitate who I am today. I am also grateful to my intimate relationships and animal friends, for creating emotionally nourishing caverns.

This book would not have been possible without the expertise of the many professionals who helped craft it, and the people who guided me during the days of turmoil, when I couldn't see the way. I'm grateful to Anand and Zubin at the Indian Art Therapy program for guiding the creative spark in me all those years ago. To the supportive mentors at the Srishti Manipal Institute of Art and Design, for opening my mind to the healing arts very young. I'm grateful to psychotherapist Beth Enterkin for taking me under her mentorship to train in sexual-violence focused trauma psychotherapy, exactly when she did, and my faculty at the School of the Art Institute of Chicago who supported my unique voice.

To Indira Bodani and the team at the Gateway School of Mumbai, for nurturing learning spaces ahead of their time, and Sarita Ganesh of the Khula Aasman Trust for trusting me with the leadership of the prison project, exactly when she did.

To the large hearts of Jehan Manekshaw and Sananda Mukhopadhyaya of Theatre Professionals, who supported innovating in arts education, and to all the spaces which pushed me to keep innovating.

To Mrs Piloo Tata and the team at the Lady Meherbai D. Tata Education Trust for supporting my clinical education, making it tangible for me to fearlessly take the uncharted path.

I feel grateful to my well-wishers at the School of the Art Institute of Chicago and the University of Michigan, where I learnt to take creative risks while expanding my lens of the field of trauma therapy.

To my publishers, HarperCollins India and my editor, Bushra, for her trust and courage in showcasing my writing as a therapeutic aid. To my agent, Ambar and the team at A Suitable Agency, for envisioning a space for my voice before I could see it.

I feel grateful to the many other unnamed people whose skills enhanced *Unashamed*'s production journey. I thank my clients profoundly for entrusting me to carry forward their life stories and helping me place them in a safe corner of the written world.

And most importantly, I thank you, the reader, for traversing this brave inner path with me. Living a heart-centred, unashamed and creative existence is one that I wish upon us all.

# Glossary

| Word/phrase | Meaning |
|---|---|
| big T trauma | experiencing or witnessing severe accidents, sexual assault, natural disasters, hate crimes, war or other situations that may have led to death. |
| buried memory | a memory or recollection that is deeply stored in one's mind and may not be readily accessible or consciously recalled. |
| collective trauma | wounding/distress caused to a group, collective or society |
| growth-oriented | an approach or mindset that prioritizes and seeks continuous progress, learning, and advancement. |
| individual trauma | wounding/distress caused to an individual human being |
| small t trauma | experiencing bullying, divorce, loss of a pet, academic stress and interpersonal conflicts that cause disruption to one's regular life. |
| trauma | a type of wounding that causes distress |

| Word/phrase | Meaning |
|---|---|
| trauma-informed | an approach or framework that recognizes that trauma is widespread and seeks to create an environment that is sensitive to and supportive of those who have experienced trauma |
| trauma response | the psychological and physiological reactions that individuals may experience in response to a traumatic event or series of events. |

# References

Scan this QR code to access the references.

# About the Author

*'Every day, from my therapy desk, I see that sexuality has been repressed in the larger Indian context. Part of my life's work is to help people normalize their own sexual expression in relationship to their personal power, to heal from sexual shame and expand their understanding of sexual trauma.'*

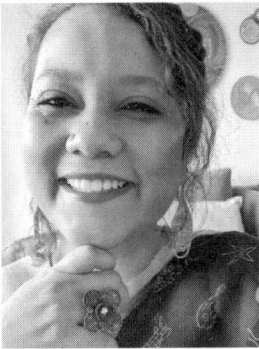

**Neha Bhat**
(ATR) Registered Art Therapist, USA
(ABT) Certified Art-based Therapy Practitioner, India
Trained Sexual Trauma Rape Crisis Counselor

Neha is a licensed sex-focused trauma psychotherapist, an artist and an educator. In her therapy practice, she uses arts-based wellness tools and principles of depth psychology while drawing from ancient Indian spiritual wisdom to assist people from diverse sociocultural backgrounds in healing the deep wounds that trauma creates, when it lives repressed within our bodies.

As a queer Indian person, making mental health practice more culturally sensitive is a key area of interest for her. Her clinic

223

is oriented towards teaching and innovation in multicultural counselling education, making inner work tools more accessible to the public. Having worked in the fields of disability education, community mental health, restorative justice, prison healthcare and sexual violence prevention at the University of Michigan, the Art Institute of Chicago, the Rush Medical Centre, St. Xavier's College and the Tata Institute of Social Sciences, she teaches therapists and healers to develop innovative solutions to navigate a complex world.

To help create more trauma-sensitive media, Neha consults on Indian films, documentaries and reality TV shows about sex and intimacy and shares free trauma psychotherapy tools as the @indiansextherapist on social media regularly.

Website: https://nehabhat.org/
Social media: @indiansextherapist (Instagram)